NATIVE AMERICAN
HERBAL
APOTHECARY

2 BOOKS IN 1

Herbalism Encyclopedia
&
Herbal Dispensatory

TAMAYA KAWISENHAWE

TABLE OF CONTENT

NATIVE AMERICAN
HERBALISM
ENCYCLOPEDIA

The forgotten secrets of medicinal
plants & their uses for healing

INTRODUCTION

The theory that underlies all medicinal, physical, and spiritual Native American healing therapies is quite basic. People must learn to live in peace with the world around them in order to live healthily. In a way, the first ecologists were Native Americans. They wanted their relationship with Mother Earth to be as harmonious as possible, and they believed that eternal stability, which was necessary for good health, would only be accomplished when they existed in harmony with the world. In recent years, it has been apparent that they were on to something. Analysis has found that our mental wellbeing influences physical fitness tremendously.

Lewis Mehl-Madrona, M.D., Medical Director of the Centre for
Complementary Medicine at the University of Pittsburgh Medical

"If we are in peace with the world and the people around us, our cells are in equilibrium inside us...Amid the difficulties she sent her way, the Native Americans sought ways of living in peace with Mother Earth." *

They committed themselves to keep all facets of their world in the highest esteem, including wild animals and poor weather. For example, when they killed a bear, they made a necklace with their teeth, worn by a warrior to honour the bravery and strength of the beast. They have often left presents such as small tobacco pouches after every good hunt to express their heartfelt thanks to Mother Earth. In the same way, they treated trees. They still did so with deep reverence, whether they cultivated plants for Medicine or fruit. They claimed that it was their way of expressing appreciation for the kindness of the Supreme Spirit, which was responsible for all living things. They claimed that a refusal to live in accordance with Mother Nature would have dire repercussions, for example, by not giving adequate thanks for good hunts and harvests. An Indian who hunted animals or gathered herbs would always sing the requisite songs or prayers or give tobacco offerings to the spirits of the animals or plants, according to one scholar, "as failure to do so could lead to sickness or bad luck." Only a few decades ago, modern ears sounded odd about this mystical approach to nature and the environment. Americans also began to see the wisdom of the holistic approach, though. The common expression "what goes around comes around" reflects how much we have come to accept the Native American way of life and respect it.

The wellness traditions and values of Native American tribes are related to Native American Medicine. Although some of these traditions exist today in some tribes, this paper looks at the issue from a historical point of view, mainly concentrating on historical sources as opposed to current traditions.
In many Native American tribes, healthcare has historically focused on the principle of harmony in every area of life. It was believed that physical, cultural, emotional, and environmental components all played a role in the wellbeing of the participant and the community. Usually, diseases are not due to physical disease alone, but rather an inconsistency in any or more of these components. As a result, many tribes claimed that both natural and spiritual causes could be the result of disease, and their medicine activities were meant to cope with both.
The tradition of Native American Medicine dates back thousands of years, but pre-European evidence of these rituals is almost non-existent since most tribes never produced a written language. Before Europeans started to gather in the 16th century in continental America, no outsiders had ever been able to capture these customs.

Furthermore, most Native American medicine practitioners at the time had no desire to share their expertise with outsiders, claiming that such experience was sacred. The adaptable, variable existence of Native American herbalism (discussed further down under Medicine) made it so that no encyclopedic medicinal works could be conveniently published to further exacerbate the matter. At that very moment, past documents of anyone's healthcare profession serve as a snapshot of an individual tribe and do not generally represent Native American Medicine as a whole. However, to recognize popular patterns and customs, these individual instances can nevertheless be observed.

The advances in medical research have had a huge effect on our lives, no doubt. Individuals enjoy fuller, happier lives than ever before. Any of the advantages of modern drugs, however, can be offset by their costs. Modern medications are pricey, not only in billions but in terms of our long-term wellbeing, maybe. That's how most operate by causing the body to answer in some ways, as powerful as medications can be, rather than by relying on the body's own natural healing forces. The body may be placed in a passive, reliant, and gradually impaired state by using medications. Remember what happens with an illness when you get it. Taking an antibiotic, which destroys the bacteria that make you sick, is the latest solution. This is a rational solution in the short term, but every day, the body is exposed to billions of bacteria. It is a losing cause in the long run. Antibiotics are just temporary protection, although essential for battling certain infections. They don't help the body improve its own defences and avoid new pathogens.

A completely new approach was taken by aboriginal healers. In their opinion, the better solutions were those that enabled the body to take care of itself instead of just offering immediate assistance. They also strongly believed in a spiritual aspect of healing that reinforced the body as well as the mind and emotions through meditation, imagination, and a number of healing rituals, making a recovery much simpler. Today, this mind-body relation is being embraced by a growing number of established practitioners. It took hundreds of years, but Native Americans' wisdom and expertise are now on the cutting edge of mainstream medical treatment.

In reality, the recent increase in "alternative" methods of healing and the use of therapeutic prayer recalls Native American methods: herbs and other so-called "natural" medicines, imagination, meditation, and more. Many individuals are shocked to discover how experienced Native Americans actually were. Mostly, in a somewhat small way, culture portrays these knowledgeable, insightful persons. Although it is accurate that Native Americans were skilled hunters, instrument-makers, and warriors, their talents were larger than that. None has been said of their remarkable skills as healers until recently. Native Americans were well-known among the early colonists for supposedly impressive curing abilities, but historians documented little of these tales, possibly owing to ethnic bias and the assumption that "savages" were Native Americans. However, reports of Native American medical prowess began to circulate by word of mouth and were reported in colonial diaries and journals. Still, we will read first-hand accounts of what the Native Americans were able to do from the early settlers.

Before Starting...

CHAPTER 1

Herbalism usually refers to traditional medicinal practice based on the use of plants and plant extracts. Herbalism is also known as phototherapy. In this chapter, we will be discussing wildcrafting, growing, and storage of herbs for Herbalism.

1.1 WILDCRAFTING

The process of collecting plants from their natural environment for nutritional or therapeutic purposes is wildcrafting. (The term 'foraging' is sometimes used, but they are synonymous, for grain and 'wildcrafting' for herbal medicines). Wildcrafted herbs can be used in a number of medicines, including tinctures, herbal salves, and infusions, and when handled mindfully, you can enjoy all the benefits of wild herbal medicines without upsetting the environment.

Wildcrafting Benefits

Wild plants, since they come from richer terrain, mostly in relatively undisturbed meadows and forests, are more potent and nutrient-dense than their monoculture counterparts. Commercial farms also have depleted soil or feed isolated nutrients to the plants only. It is a perfect way to experience the outdoors as well. For a relaxing expedition, you should bring a mate. And there are many easy herbal remedies you can make with your harvest of wild plants when you return home.

WILDCRAFTING HERBS WILL HELP YOUR EFFORTS TO:

Eat foods that are nutrient-dense
Reduce reliance on imported medicines and food
Decrease reliance on Major Agro
Experience and enjoy nature

With natural tonics & remedies, keep yourself healthy! At the same time, you can also bring family and friends along and build a community.

What to bring when you're going wildcrafting:

You don't really need a lot of equipment, but there are a few essentials that can really make your journey a smooth one. You're going to need something mostly to bring your harvest in, and you may need some instruments to distinguish the plants from the forest.

For short journeys, baskets are great, and for longer ones, big paper bags are great. Don't store herbs in plastic because they can decompose quickly in the sun. You would need something for slicing, digging and snipping, depending on what you want to harvest. If you're digging roots, you'll want a trowel, and if you have to hack bark or roots, bring a decent knife, and some kitchen shears or scissors for snipping greenery or flowers.

For all kinds of wildcrafting and gardening duties, I love this Hori digging knife. It has one smooth blade and one serrated blade and it is angled so that it acts as a knife and a trowel. A vegetable brush is another handy tool to clean roots with, to reduce the dirt you take with you. Carry a paintbrush instead of a crop brush if you're picking mushrooms to avoid destroying them.

1.2. SITE SELECTION

Obtaining permission: On BLM property, if you receive limited sums, a free use permit can be received for a low fee. The U.S. Both Forest Service and BLM will warn you that there is no picking (a) in or near campgrounds or picnic areas; (b) some trails less than 200 feet away; and (c) on the side of the lane.

1. Keep away from downwind runoff, roadsides (at least 50 feet), electric high-voltage cables (may cause mutations), lawn and public park fertilizers, downstream mines or agribusiness, near parking lots, and even spray areas. Routine spraying is used by several BLM and Forest Service areas. This also refers to private property, where you would need to worry about herbicides and pesticides.

2. A reckless wildcrafter will seriously alter a rocky hillside or stream-side habitat using discretion in vulnerable ecosystems.

1.3. GROWING AND PROPAGATION TECHNIQUES

1. Using proper techniques for wild crafts can ensure minimal effects, improve harvest yields, and help to provide wildlife with plant food. Year after year, do not harvest the same stand but tend the field as needed. Techniques used for "gardening" include thinning, root separation, top pinching, and protection of a wide variety of grandparent plants to seed and protect young plants.

2. Be mindful of conditions contributing to erosion. Replant or disperse seeds if digging roots and close gaps. Be conscious of stands on the hillside, add vegetation and soil around areas cleared. It could be appropriate to gather foliage from surrounding collected plants and scatter it around. Wearing hard-soled shoes can inflict irreparable harm to fragile hillside ecosystems.

3. Don't pull the roots while extracting the leaves. Root yields, as well as foliage, can be improved by flower pruning of some species.

4. Allow seasonal findings on areas produced by wildlife. Be mindful of your harvested stands and check the various cycles of growth. This will measure the true effect on the Environment. (An established wild crafter in the northwest has found that a stable population would rise by around 30% a year once it enters stasis. Anything less than this may be called degenerative.)

1.4. SUGGESTED GATHERING TIMES

1. Aerial or above-ground parts: from 6 to 10 a.m. in the mornings, just until they wilt in the light. Some are stronger just before flowering when collecting leaves.

2. You should be able to see the bud's colour by picking most flowers only before they are starting to bloom. Around or after the full moon is the typical moon period for collecting aerial parts.

3. **Roots:** Harvest after seeding; early in the morning, if possible, before the sun reaches. Biennials: harvest in the first year's fall or the second year's season. A new moon is a conventional period.

4. **Barks**: In the spring or autumn, harvest. Don't strip ever. Take a whole crop. In dense cities, tree thinning is acceptable, but the healthiest looking trees still leave. Be mindful of potentially leaving the tree vulnerable to fungal rot if you take only from the small branches. The inner bark, or cambium, is the most active bark of many, for pollarding, leaving short trunks and low stumps for coppicing. This will supply a continuous production. The typical bark process is three-quarters of the waning light.

5. **Saps & Pitches**: Late winter or early spring harvest.

6. **Seed & Fruit**: Harvest when ripe, with some variations, such as oranges, unripe pods of scarlet beans, etc.

1.5. DRYING

1. Dry most plants in shaded, well-ventilated areas; avoid wire screens and newspaper print. Research which plants dry better in the sun.

2. Don't wash the flowers or plants. Shake them to clear off pests and ashes. Where amounts are reasonable, tie bundles with diameters of 1 1/2 inches or less at the stems' base. They can also be loosely dispersed to dry on windows.

3. Barks: If possible, peel the outer bark off. It's called tossing here.

4. Roots: Spread out or loop them. Usually, rinsing won't dissolve soil particles. As well as hand brushing, particularly with clay, a pressure hose is often needed. For broad, heavy roots without aromatic properties, cut lengthwise.

5. When fragile, all plant components are dry. Pinch the hanging plants in the lower section. To see if the core is dry, cut a large sample root in half.

TO PRODUCE INFUSIONS OF HOT WATER

Leaves:
1 ounce per quart of water, 4 hours in hot water, securely sealed.
Tougher leaves need steeping for longer.

Flowers:
1 ounce per quart of water, in hot water for 2 hours.
Less time is needed for more delicate flowers.

Seeds:
1 ounce per pint of water, in hot water for 30 minutes.
Less time is required for more fragrant seeds such as fennel (15 minutes),
longer rose hips (3 to 4 hours).

Barks & Roots:
1 ounce per pint of water, in hot water for 8 hours.
Less (1 to 2 hours) for certain barks,
such as slippery elm.

1.6. STORAGE

1. Stop heat that is light and excessive and might kill aromatic properties and other important constituents. Food grade plastic bags or fiber barrels or other containers that emit oxygen and moisture are suitable to retain consistency and potency as long as possible while they are completely dry.

2. Mark with place and dates.

3. Broken or crushed herbs lose their worth more easily than uncut herbs, which are complete.

The Rocky Mountain Herbalists' Group has established approaches to conserving wild medicinal plant species. Deep feelings for the sanctity of the Environment and plant communities are the impetus for developing these methods. As a non-governmental group operating in a single bioregion, these techniques are structured to include informed self-interest and social coercion. These methods are available for use, modified, and implemented to their own unique needs by those in other bioregions.

The first move was to establish a series of rules to help harvesters grasp the core concepts of ethical wildlife crafting. With many experienced wildcrafters' feedback, these standards have been established and submitted to rigorous peer review. Instead of being hard and fast guidelines, they are built to compliment the ethical framework. For the wildcrafter to fill out and submit along with each shipment of herbs, a requirements sheet containing details on where and how a plant is grown, handled, and dried has been produced. This data offers customers the ability to learn about responsible wildlife crafting and explicitly help harvesters whose philosophies are in line with their own.

The next move was to establish a list of conscientious wild craftsmen and organic farmers for direct marketing. By placing herb buyers in line with the actual harvesters, the register was designed to promote good actions. This direct connection promotes an atmosphere of shared interest, helps improve quality management, and encourages wildcrafters to set rates that enhance sustainable harvesting practices and inspire them.

Manufacturers of herbal products are encouraged to use the list to integrate the values into their routine business activities. Wild crafters and organic farmers who are ecologically conscious are invited to send additional listings to the new register. The development of a bio-regional cooperative of wild craftsmen and organic farmers is a recent phase in this initiative.

The concept is to come together as a group to share information; encourage education among harvesters and growers; establish self-regulation systems by peer review; and meet demands at a price that promotes healthy, ecologically sound practices for ethically harvested and organically grown herbs. The co-op is a vehicle for participants to exchange knowledge about plant growth patterns, harvesting procedures, methods of propagation and production, and alternatives to over-harvesting. A list of native plants that are threatened, threatened, over-cultivated, or illegally cultivated is being established, and restrictions are set to ensure species' survival by peer consensus.

This knowledge can be shared in a newsletter with other wildcrafters, bio-regional co-ops, and customers. It is also possible to establish a seed sharing scheme so that regions can be re-seeded for potential use. For the co-op, to ensure that some areas are not overused and that other regions are left behind to regenerate, participants will be able to exchange knowledge on harvesting regions. The cooperative aims to create a system that can be used to direct each other and develop personal honesty. In order to protect areas from forestry, construction, and agriculture, the co-op may also be seen as a forum for citizens to work together as activists. We would like to see the development of an annual meeting where wild craftsmen can meet, exchange data, reinforce the network, and become a prominent, active member of the herbal culture.

There is an urgency for those who hear the sound of the Earth weeping, Herbalist or not, to do something to respond. This is a start to secure and help this tiny portion of the planet survive. The Rocky Mountain Herbalists' Alliance insists that we must be careful not to kill wild plant species or the wild places where they live either directly through our own acts or implicitly through our implicit agreement. To do this, we need to take precautions to put long-term survival at the grassroots and corporate level before short-term gain. If we take a stand together and stick to ethical values, those who disregard the plants will either change their processing methods or vanish from the sector. In this way, we seek to undo the harm done by our forebears, retain our own sacred faith in the World, and give our descendants the gift of respect for life seen on stable and prosperous earth.

1.7. HERBAL PREPARATIONS: MAKING INFUSIONS AND DECOCTIONS

An infusion is made by immersing an herb in either cold or hot (not boiling) water. The stream, not drinking water, can be the purest you can find. It is safer to provide water from rainfall, good wells or streams, or bottled water. Herbs with potent volatile oils are better infused in cold water (those with a clear scent like essential oil or perfume). In warm water, some herbs perform well. Depending on the plant, they can be left for a period of time, from fifteen minutes to overnight, so that the water will consume the plant's basic elements. For the production of infusions and decoctions, glass or earthenware vessels are great. As they won't crack from fire, quart or pint canning jars are fine, and the screw cap prevents the nutrients from floating away in the steam.

An Example Of A Hot Infusion

This infusion is used because of its general nutritional properties, especially for menopausal women. For anyone weighing 130 to 160 pounds, the rule-of-thumb is to take an infusion of 16 ounces (2 cups) every day.

1. Mix together the dried, sliced, and sifted nettles, oat-straw, red clover, alfalfa, horsetail, and spearmint for one pound each.
2. Place one cup of the mixture in a quart pot, fill it with hot water, and screw on the lid.
3. Just quit overnight.
4. Strain the mixture in the morning to extract all the ingredients and then drink it for the next two days. As they tend to go poor, do not keep infusions for more than two days.

For herbs, which work differently in cold and hot water, cold infusions are preferable. Yarrow, for example, when cooked in hot water, can be very bitter, but when cooked in cold water, it is not bitter. Yarrow's aromatic components, and their associated antispasmodic properties, are soluble in cold water, while the herb's acidic components are not. Cool infusions are formulated the same way as hot infusions, but a time span unique to itself would need to be soaked in each herb. This can only be learned over time, while several herbal books on the market can offer advice. Prepared with hot water, decoctions can be far more potent than infusions. In three cups of water, the general procedure is to slowly take one ounce of herb and simmer slowly until the liquid decreases by half. Use just a bottle made of stainless steel or glass, never aluminium. Depending on the plant employed, the dosages will vary from a tablespoon to a cup. The decoctions should be kept refrigerated for a period of two days only.

Tincturing Herbs

A tincture for internal use is made by immersing a fresh or dry plant in either straight alcohol or an alcohol and water mixture. Plants produce a certain amount of water when young, naturally. A fresh herb, one part of an herb per two parts of alcohol, is put in 190-proof alcohol (95 percent alcohol). If you had three ounces (dry measure) of fresh yarrow, for example, it would be placed in a container of 190-proof alcohol with six ounces (liquid measure), Mason jars are really good. The cap is screwed on, and the tincture is kept out of the heat for two weeks. It is decanted at the end of the duration, and the herb is pressed onto a rag to extract as much moisture as possible. Alcohol sucks all the water it absorbs out of a plant. A combination of both water and alcohol would be the resultant tincture. While many herbalists do so with fresh herbs, I do not cut or chop them into small bits. They assume that the heavier the tincture, the greater the surface area that is subjected to the alcohol. The herbs like to be kept whole in my job. We seldom develop fresh tincture roots. We cut them into smaller pieces as we do so. We still leave as whole as we can while tincturing the above-ground plant stuff. Each person must learn what works best. Plants lose their natural moisture content when they mature. There are tables on the moisture content of many medicinal plants available. Michael Moore, from his Southwest School of Botanical Medicine, gives a strong one. Certain plants have almost nothing, such as myrrh gum, and others have plenty of water, such as mint. When you make a dry plant tincture, the amount of water that was present in the plant when it was fresh is added back into the mixture. Dried plants are typically tinctured at a five-to-one ratio; that is, five liquid pieces to one dried herb part. The Osha root, for example, contains 30 percent water by weight. You'd apply fifty ounces of liquid, 35 ounces of 95% alcohol, and 15 ounces of water to it if you had ten ounces of powdered Osha core. You don't want to use drinking water ever since freshwater is a must.

As a general rule, dried herbs are powdered as thinly as possible, often in a blender. Until they are required, it is best to store them whole. Again, the tincture is left for two weeks and then decanted, and the medicinal content is squeezed out of the oil. For new seeds, you will normally pull as many out as you put in. You get out as much as you can with dry stuff, specifically roots. As they shield the tincture's purity from the chemical deterioration that can result from sunlight, amber jars are useful for tincture preservation. So safe, several years will last for the tinctures. For dispensing, herbal tinctures should then be mixed together (though a few do not mix well). Many herbalists choose tinctures because of their long-lasting consistency and ease of dispensing. In several herbal texts, dosages for tinctures are included.

TINCTURE FORMULA FOR UPSET STOMACH AND NAUSEA

Ten millilitres each of yarrow, poleo mint (or peppermint), and betony
Place in a one-ounce amber bottle with dropper
Take 1/3 to 1/2 dropper as needed

Making Oil Infusions For Salves

The first part of making a salve is to transfer the plant's medicinal properties to an oil base. Then the oil is made thick and moderately hard by the addition of beeswax. To make an oil infusion of dried herbs, grind the herbs you wish to use into as fine a powder as possible. Place the ground herbs in a glass baking dish and cover with oil. Olive oil is a good choice. Stir the herbs to make sure they are well saturated with oil and then add enough oil to cover them by 1/2 to 1/4 inch. Cook them in the oven on low heat for eight hours (overnight). Some herbalists prefer to cook the herbs as long as ten days at 100 degrees. When ready, strain the herbs' oil by pressing in a strong cloth with a good weave. To make an oil infusion from fresh herbs, place the herbs in a mason jar, and cover them with just enough oil to make sure that no part of the plant is exposed to air. Let sit in the sun for two weeks. Then press the herbs through a cloth. Let the decanted oil sit. After a day, the water, naturally present in the herbs, will settle to the bottom. Pour off the oil and discard the water. Some herbalists prefer to start the oil infusion by letting the herb sit for 24 hours in just a bit of alcohol that has been poured over the leaves. They then add the oil and allow it to stand for two weeks. The water and alcohol remain behind when the oil is poured off.

1.8. USEFUL INFORMATION ABOUT HERBALISM

In many ways, you can learn about herbs. Teachers who exchange experiences and practical information are one of the best opportunities to understand. They will have keen insights into herbs and their applications. Find educators who follow the ancient methods of herbal medicine within your culture. Take a lesson or workshop, or work on a farm with plants. To receive insights on how to manage the plants, form a mentoring relationship. It is also important that the plants spend time with you. Pick a plant that grows in your yard or sit down with a cup of herbal tea outdoors.

What are you seeing?
What is it that smells like?
How does it make you feel when you drink
tea made from grass?

Your experience is incomplete until you've spent time feeling, hearing, smelling, and eating the herb. And then you may, of course, check the many books on herbs and Herbalism which are available. We are lucky to have access to books written years ago and to books written since then for centuries. They include multiple facets and factors of herbal medicine (such as astrology), and most agree on the plant should be used where and how each one is used. This expertise was derived from years of analysis, training, and practice. However, once in a while, you can find data that varies from what you have heard elsewhere in one source. With the diverse viewpoints they often discover when they study herbs, I try to find fun in my students' desperation. This is a positive thing, though! Each Herbalist gives a thorough account of his or her own experience with the herb and how it functions. This knowledge is the product of the Herbalist's interaction with the plant. For the same leaf, you might have a slightly different experience, and that is good. Several herbal practitioners can agree that when they are eaten, herbs have unique purposes. Herbs help remove waste from the body. If the body undergoes slow digestion or insufficient detoxification, herbs move the old to make room for the fresh. Herbs facilitate recovery. Their vitamins and minerals intake help the body to regenerate and recover normal structure and function. In the body, herbs increase overall energy. Herbs offer a reinforcement that helps cure and detoxify the body, which raises the vitality levels of everyday life.

This book is for the herbal lover, who is searching for a lot of data in one location at the outset. Many herbal books concentrate on particular herbs, medication, or herbal history, but I decided to write a book with a little bit of both, both from a conventional and a science point of view. I am a gatherer of knowledge as a herbalist and biochemist, and naturopathic practitioner. My effort to share some of what I have heard about herbs in this book. In a metaphysical, science, and conventional way, I hope its components can help you understand herbal medicine. I have given the knowledge that I hope will help you interpret this complex method from a holistic viewpoint by mixing together anatomy, plant definitions, and herbal therapy concepts to develop a clearer understanding of how and when to use plants as medicine.

Remember that traditional Herbalism is much more complicated than what is described in this book when you begin your herbal studies. Herbalism focuses on a broader basis that incorporates the principles of tissue conditions (excitement, depression, atrophy, stagnation, anxiety, relaxation), the four characteristics of the plant (hot, cold, dry, damp), the disposition of the consumer, and the vitality (the subtle energies). We may not even know how herbs work as medicine, but there are several philosophies. However, we know that they act to manage whole body processes in a systemic manner rather than a single symptom. They nourish and maintain equilibrium in the body such that disharmonious organs will return to full operation. As a plant is introduced into the body, at a cellular stage, it is recognized. The body recognizes the constituents of the plant and appears to understand how to break them down and bring them to function where they are needed. While herbs can be beneficial at many physiological dimensions and measures, they work first with the body to identify and care for the region in greatest need. We can also get imaginative with preparation, mixing different herbs into formulations that concentrate with a much greater aim.

Many herbs are rich in minerals that supply the body with the required healing components to promote cell regeneration, digestion, digestion, and heart functionality. After herbs are administered to demonstrate their efficacy, we may clinically evaluate their physiological function. List some cases. Ginger produces very strong compounds called gingerols, which are anti-inflammatory. Several clinical trials involving patients with arthritis showed that ginger extracts influenced the inflammatory mechanism at the cellular level to alleviate discomfort and inflammation. Blood cell counts assessed following immune-stimulating herb administration indicate elevated amounts of white cells. Good improvements in cellular structure have been seen by biopsies obtained during herbal administration. Modern medicine has done an outstanding job in isolating plants and body elements, but the complex concepts in holism and structural harmony are seriously absent. Be mindful of the entire structure rather than the particular parts or signs, whether you are contemplating a plant or the body.

When you use herbs, think in a holistic way about the whole plant and how it can affect the body. Meadowsweet tea, for instance, is often used to cure problems with the stomach and can be especially effective for children with diarrhoea. Salicylic acid, which is an essential ingredient in aspirin, is one constituent (a chemically active portion within the herb) of meadowsweet. If salicylic acid is swallowed in an isolated way, the stomach wall can become irritated. But meadowsweet contains antioxidants called polyphenols, in addition to salicylic acid, that protect the stomach wall. This ensures that the desired behaviour of pain relief is provided by meadowsweet without the side effect of stomach discomfort.

I never see a patient in my office who is facing a problem in isolation. It is possible that other systems or organs are still failing when one system or organ is struggling. We ought to remember some significant points when we use herbs when we incorporate this way of thought to heal the body from a holistic viewpoint. Identify the trigger and handle it. While acute cases, such as burns, can often be rapidly soothed with herbs, study and the fostering of equilibrium within all body systems are necessary for long-standing disharmony. Look at the body as a whole. What physical pain do you consider normal? What signs have you endured for so long that they are almost no longer noticed by you? We may become detached from what is happening in our bodies and the symptoms and signals of pain in the hustle and bustle of our busy lives. Trust in nature's strength. Take a look around, and you can find that everywhere there are medicinal plants. Many plants that thrive in some regions are unique to the treatment of that region's diseases. For example, where I live in the Pacific Northwest, rosemary and cedar plants grow in abundance.

Vintage illustration #1_Cedar Cones

For our ever-present humid conditions, which can damage the respiratory tract and joints, all are fantastic. The secret is avoidance. Don't fool yourself that you should live and do little but support a long and stable life. Treat it gently, consider the signs of pain and symptoms, and learn how to support it as it talks to you. I am glad to be a part of it where you are on your herbal trip. Speaking from experience, I know that knowing a medicinal plant and using it to make you feel better will transform lives.

Go slowly through the book to digest and re-read all that is found inside it many times to cement these ideas for learning forever. Get out between the plants, they're the best coaches. I hope you can use this book as a practical aid and see it as a gateway to a more holistic way of living and healing. Teach and share with others and teach yourself. Reclaim the details that once were openly shared by all.

The Way Of Herbalist

Plant medicine was widely taught in households at one time, throughout the Americas and elsewhere, and circulated among societies. While the growth of modern medicine has contributed to a decline in these methods, the use of herbal medicine is causing a mass revival in North America at least, and herbal practitioners are leading others through the magic and practicality of herbal control.

The origins of herbal medicine are hard to trace, but we know that indigenous cultures have used medicinal plants for many centuries. Originally, herbs were consumed as common ingredients, but human interest being what it is, some time and energy spent on experimenting with plants and started to understand their health and healing importance.

Herbs have been used for weakness and fever, broken bones, blood infections, and many other disorders since ancient times. Eventually, people accepted that herbs' protective use appeared to encourage some of their best effects, reinforcing the body to combat disease. The vinegar of the four thieves, drunk during the bubonic plague outbreak by robbers from Marseilles, France, is one such example. None of the robbers who took frequent injections of the vinegar succumbed to the plague after plundering the houses of those who had fallen ill. At one time, medicinal herbs, like basic herbs known for their ability to relieve fever, cure wounds, and treat bites, were mostly cultivated in home gardens.

Herbal remedies were widespread, and he might go to a house where rosemary grew if a person did not know the right herb to cure an illness, thinking this would be the place to get herbal knowledge. Herbal cures were exchanged as information was handed on from generation to generation, just like sharing any good story. In fact, many of our grandmothers cooked herbal concoctions and stored them in the closet.

Herbal remedies started to be mistrusted as inferior medicine at some level when the era of industrial medicine grew, not because they were unhealthy or dangerous, but because they were deemed inferior to the new prescription drugs. You have a lot to think and something to be enthusiastic about as an aspiring herbalist. I've spoken about their interest in herbs and why it started with countless people. It was a basic recognition for everyone that what was being presented regarding herbs' medicinal usage appeared to make a great deal of sense. Herbal medicine offered something soothing and calming, unlike the sometimes daunting and confounding American model of western medicine. I like to believe that learning the principles of herbs and how they work gives us faith that we can take care of ourselves and our loved ones responsibly whether our family members or we suffer a cold or flu, a disturbed tummy, or a muscle strain, for example. The relationship built between the human and the plants is one aspect of herbs that I really enjoy. Each journey is distinct, and plant medicine supports it, providing countless support and creating knowledge and skill ties.

Research and herbal medicine

German-Swiss physicist and alchemist Paracelsus and Herbalist, physician, and astrologer Nicholas Culpepper developed the medicine of botanical plants, mathematics, and alchemy, and astrology in the sixteenth and seventeenth centuries. While in the present day, the naturopathic elements of botany and mathematics have been brought to legitimized occupations, astrology and alchemy appear to others to be mere superstition. But to build a balanced method of studying, understanding, and using plant medicine in inconsistent ways, this mixture of studies is required. Scientific research today has helped us explore plants, their properties, and how they act when used as herbal medicines.

Herbal treatments have been checked and proven time and time again to produce the same outcomes. Many herbs have been researched extensively, and there is no doubt that they do have healing properties and that they are powerful and healthy. Herbal science and legislation are hot topics, and I'm not strong in my position on these issues, truth be told. However, research can help further the use of plant remedies and inform and encourage knowledge of herbs' healing properties. I deal with the general public, and my herb shop is visited every day by a wide spectrum of people, from those who know little about herbs to professionally qualified herbalists. Any individuals need a clinical understanding of how plants function inside the body, and they are suspicious of natural treatments without this. Perhaps further study will open the doors for those who are less able by traditional approaches to learning about herbs. It's necessary to note that not all experiments are accurate. Still, look for specifics of some analysis you read. Who did the test? On one part of the plant or the whole thing, was the test performed? Will the researcher make or sell a product relevant to the test that is marketed? Depending on its intentions, this knowledge may give good guidance as to whether the examination is factual or subjective. If you wish to advance your herbal research interests, I suggest the American Botanical Council (abc.herbalgram.org) and the work of its president, herbalist Mark Blumenthal.

1.10. SAFETY TIPS – USE AND ABUSE OF HERBS

German-Swiss physicist and alchemist Paracelsus and Herbalist, physician, and astrologer Nicholas Culpepper developed the positions in medicine of botanical plants, mathematics, alchemy, and astrology in the sixteenth and seventeenth centuries. While in the present day, the naturopathic elements of botany and mathematics have been brought to legitimized occupations, astrology and alchemy appear to others to be mere superstition. But to build a balanced method of studying, understanding, and using plant medicine in inconsistent ways, this mixture

1.9. HERBS SHOPPING GUIDE

Lingle's Herbs
2055 N. Lomina Avenue
Long beach, CA 90815
800-708-0633
Organically grown herbal plant

Jean's Herbal Tea Works
119 Sulphur Springs Road
Norway, NY 13416
888-845-TEAS
www.jeansgreen.com

Medicinal Herbal Teas
Glenbrook Farm herbs and Such
1538 Shiloh Road
Campbellsville, KY 42718
888-716-7627
www.glenbrookfarm.com/herbs
Nonirradiated herbs and herbal
products

Well Sweep Herbal Farm
205 Mt. Bethel Road
Port Murray, NJ 07865
008-852-5390
www.wellsweep.com
High quality herbal plants

Vitamin Express
1-800-500-0733
www.vitaminexpress.com
herbs, herbal extracts, vitamins,
minerals and
performance supplements

Blessed Herbs
109 Barre Plains Road
Oakham, MA 01068
800-489-4372
www.blessedherbs.com
Mail-order herbs

Maitake Products, Inc.
222 Bergen Turnike
Ridgefield park, NJ 07660
800-747-7418
www.maitake.com
Mail-order herbs

Dry Creek Herbs Farm
10121 Wolf Road
Grass valley, CA 95945
888-489-8454
Organically grown herbs

of studies is required. Scientific research today has helped us explore plants, their properties, and how they act when used as herbal medicines. Herbal treatments have been checked and proven time and time again to produce the same outcomes. Many herbs have been researched extensively, and there is no doubt that they do have healing properties and that they are powerful and healthy.

Herbal science and legislation are hot topics, and I'm not strong in my position on these issues, truth be told. However, research can help further the use of plant remedies and inform and encourage knowledge of herbs' healing properties. I deal with the general public, and my herb shop is visited every day by a wide spectrum of people, from those who know little about herbs to professionally qualified herbalists. Any individuals need a clinical understanding of how plants function inside the body, and they are suspicious of natural treatments without this. Perhaps further study will open the doors for those who are less able by traditional approaches to learning about herbs. It's necessary to note that not all experiments are accurate. Still, look for specifics of some analysis you read. Who did the test? On one part of the plant or the whole thing, was the test performed? Will the researcher make or sell a product relevant to the test that is marketed? Depending on its intentions, this knowledge may give good guidance as to whether the examination is factual or subjective. If you wish to advance your herbal research interests, I suggest the American Botanical Council (abc.herbalgram.org) and the work of its president, herbalist Mark Blumenthal.

1.11. ESSENTIAL TOOLS

Aluminium foil
Baking dish
Calculator
Cheesecloth
Coffee filters
Coffee or nut grinder
Cooking brush or paintbrush
Cooking thermometer
Crockpot
Fine mesh strainers, small, medium, and large
Funnels, small, medium, and large
Glass containers, quart-size with secure lids
Mason jars, pint and quart size
Measuring cups, small, medium, and large
Mixing bowls
Mixing spoons
Muddling bar
Notebook
Packing rod
Pencil
Percolation vessel
Plastic sandwich bags
Rocks or paperweights
Rubber bands
Saucepan, stainless steel or ceramic
Shot glass
Soaking basin
Stockpot, stainless steel or ceramic
Vitamix blender
Waxed paper

1.12. FORAGING & HARVESTING

Growing your own herbs at home is an amazing way to enjoy fresh flavours all year long. And as the weather starts turning cooler and the days get shorter, that just means one thing: its harvest time!
There are a few things you should keep in mind when harvesting herbs, no matter what herb you're harvesting.

Here's some practical advice:

- Only pick herbs when they're dry.
- It is advisable to harvest after the morning dew has evaporated, or at dusk.
- Harvest culinary herbs just before the buds open.
- Be sure to pinch any buds before they flower because once they bloom, all the plant's energy goes into producing blooms, and thus the tasty leaves don't develop well.
- Harvest seeds before they turn from green to brown.
- Seeds must not be brown but brittle, dry, and crushable, be gentle!
- When you harvest, handle them with care to avoid bruising your precious harvest as fresh herbs are fragile, so.

Sustainable Foraging Guidelines

1. Only forage abundant plants with a large, widespread population. Never harvest a plant without first analysing its population and the threats of habitat destruction or commercial demand that it could face. For example, a plant can be locally abundant, but if there is widespread demand, it will easily vanish, with overharvesting decimating its population.

2. Favour harvesting plants that are non native. Whether a plant is native and bound to local food chains or is an escapee from other lands is one of the first things I remember when selecting which plants to forage. By vying with them for natural resources, non natives displace native animals. With the same checks and balances that natural plants have encountered, these opportunistic plants have not evolved locally, and so they often thrive. This makes them

prime forage for us humans, especially because they stay close to places we occupy, flourishing in towns, gardens, fields, and the like. Many of our more popular wild weedy medicinal items are non-natives in the south eastern United States, including multiflora rose (Rosa multiflora), Japanese honeysuckle (Lonicera japonica), mimosa (Albizia julibrissin), burdock (Arctium minus), and many blackberry and raspberry species (Rubus spp.).

3. Tend the spaces "in between". Wild weeds will inevitably appear and make themselves at home with those of you who cultivate a greenhouse and will cohabit happily with cultivated vegetables and herbs. You can use lots of tricks to make them play fair, and you'll reap even more food and medicine from your garden as a reward for serving as a botanical referee! This is the bounty that rises in between the medicine and vegetables you haven't cultivated yet that you already have to harvest. My plant friend Frank Cook, who died, used to teach in his classes that in the shape of useful opportunistic plants, more than half of the bounty of a garden could be found in the "in between." In this plentiful resource, people all over the world capitalize, casually "cultivating" weeds in the in-between areas. As an example of this useful-weed-and-planted-crop-polyculture process, let's take lamb's quarters. Lamb quarters contain more nutrition, beta-carotene, vitamin C, zinc, and calcium than cultivated spinach, also called wild spinach. Why would you root out such a healthy plant that does not require special treatment or pest protection to make way for less healthy crops and more difficult to grow?

4. Only be a steward. And when you pick ample (possibly pesky) seeds, adhere to a code of ethics. After all, you're dealing with living, breathing people. Take just what you need, leave your wake with beauty (leave no trace), and carry an offer to make a song, some water, your hair, a handful of grain before you go. An offering invites a sense of respect, reciprocity, and reverence. If you're more science-minded, you could take a moment to consciously breathe, meditating on the reciprocity of the exchange of plant-human oxygen, cellular respiration, and photosynthesis. At first, you may feel stupid, but give yourself the chance to be shocked. This is how the ancient plant-human dance

of reciprocal relation, contact, and caring affects us. Be particularly careful about not overharvesting if the plant you're harvesting is organic, and you've already assessed that it's plentiful enough to grow. If you're picking a multi-stem herbaceous plant, take out a stem or two from each plant. Spread the crop over a wider field to make sure you leave plants with plenty of flowers and fruit to reproduce. Replant the root crown while you're extracting roots or take just a portion of the root system of each plant. Be careful to cut back the aboveground sections while digging up roots so that the plant does not become overwhelmed by water with a root system that no longer suits its aboveground growth. For resistant weeds with worldwide spread, these regenerative methods don't really need to be pursued.

5. Harvesting in fields where you know no one has herbicide sprayed. As the surrounding soil is usually polluted with lead, herbicides, and other pollutants, it is necessary to avoid cultivating plants near highways, railroads, and power lines. Typically farm at least 30 feet from the road and make sure you do not farm in an environmentally hazardous area (such as a dirty river flood bank). Herbicides can be applied to even hay fields Often troublesome are the foundations of older buildings since they are usually sprayed for pest protection or weeds. Try visiting a nearby organic urban farm or community garden if you live in the city, where you can possibly encounter an array of tasty vegetables, along with gardeners who are eager to share the harvest.

Native American Herbs

CHAPTER 2

2.1. ALOE - *Aloe Doctrina*

Family: *Asphodelaceae*

Popular names: Mumbai aloe, turkey aloe, Zanzibar aloe, mocha aloe.

Botanical Name:

Features: Aloe, a genus of almost two hundred species of succulent plants of mainly South African descent. The properties of this plant were known to the ancient Greeks, and for more than two thousand years, it was collected at Socotra. Aloe thrives in warm regions, and in Florida, it grows wild. In form, it is just like a succulent cactus. The leaves are generally elongated, deep brown or olive, some-times pointy, blunt or spiny-toothed, blotched, or mottled at times. The stem, with a basal rosette of leaves, is usually short.

Taste: quirky and sour. Powder: shiny yellow. The tubular red or yellow flowers are contained in simple or branched clusters on a stem. In the various varieties, these properties change slightly, with certain species becoming tree-like with forked roots. Aloe bainesii is 15 feet thick at the base and rises to heights of 65 feet. Like the miniature ones grown in homes, other varieties of Aloe are often cultivated in succulent gardens; they require bright light and diligent watering. The "American Aloe" is not an Aloe, but an American Agave.

Medicinal Part: A greenish, transparent, salve-like material, the insipid juice of the leaves.

Solvent: With water.

Bodily Influence: Emmenagogue, tonic, purgative, anthelmintic.

Uses: Among natural remedies, Aloe is one of the most sovereign agents we have, cleaning the morbid matter of the stomach, liver, spleen, kidney, and bladder. In breastfeeding, or when one suffers from haemorrhoids, Aloe may never be used alone, as in haemorrhoids, it excites and irritates the lower intestine—widely used in menstruation reduction, dyspepsia, skin lesions, liver disease, headaches, etc.

Dose: 1/2-2 grains, depending on age and disease, in powder form, for constipation; 5-10 grains twice daily for obstructed or suppressed menstruation. To kill threadworms, dissolve the Aloe in warm water and use as an injection. It is possible to take the same blend internally for multiple days.

Note: Due to the disagreeable flavour, powdered Aloe made into a solid decoction and rubbed over the nipples will help wean a breastfeeding infant. For external usage, Aloe demonstrates the same cleansing ability. When a strip of white linen or cotton soaked with aloe water is applied, fresh wounds, as well as old ones, are easily covered. Sprinkle aloe powder thick enough to cover the open wound and seal it with clean gauze if ulcers move to a running level, repeated regularly. The powder would consume the morbid, liquid matter while supporting safe new replacement tissue at the same time. For tender sunburns, bug bites, over-exposure to X-ray or other emollient requirements, the fresh juice, or formula made from dried herbs, is relaxing. In radio and X-ray skincare, it is necessary to note that aloe leaves prepared with castor oil or eucalyptus oil are curing agents and moisturizers to avoid further complications.

Caution: Should not give during menstruation or breastfeeding, or for stacks, in cases of degeneration of the liver and gallbladder. As a general, Aloe is safe to use as it is developed by folk medicine, but guidance from qualified or skilled professionals in this field should be obtained in all complicated situations.

2.2. ARSESMART - *Polygonum Hydropiper*

Family: *Polygonaceae*

Common Names: The water pepper is called hot arsesmart. Since the leaves are much like the leaves of a peach tree, also called plumbago, the mild arsesmart is called dead arssmare or peach work.

Features: A well-known plant in America that grows in the lowlands and on streams that are dry in most areas of the year. In the late summer or early autumn, its flowers, and in August, the seeds are ripe. If the split-leaf is touched to the lips, the arsesmart plants are similar, and they all have a hot feeling. The mild water pepper has much wider leaves when viewed together. They are used collectively by most herbalists. The leaves contain essential oils, oxymethylene-anthraquinones, and polygonic acid with irritant effects, glycoside, which facilitates blood coagulation, and ethereal oil containing polygonone, which decreases blood pressure. The plant contains formic acid, baldric acid, acetic acid, plenty of tannins, and a small amount of essential oil. When brought into contact with the nostrils or eyes, the fresh plant generates an acrid juice that induces itching and smarting. As in the case of mustard poultice, the bruised leaves, as well as the seeds, can raise blisters if used as a poultice.

Medicinal part: The herb in its entirety.

Solvents: Tobacco, water.

Bodily influence: Diaphoretic, stimulant, diuretic.

Uses: Effective for putrid ulcers in humans and animals (internal and external), with cooling and drying consistency. When the juice or the fractured plant is added, broken cuts, fractures, joint felons, or congealed blood may dissolve. Cold tea kills worms and cleanses the rot. Dilute tincture that is lowered in the ears removes worms in it. The bruised root or seeds placed on an aching tooth will ease the pain.

Dose: One teaspoonful of small or granulated herb split into one cup of boiling water; one cup of the cold drink through the day, one cup of mouthwash at a time. 30–60 drops of tincture.

2.3. BITTERROOT - *Apocynum Androsaemifolium*

Family: *Apocynaceae*

Common Names: Dogbane, Westernwall, Milkweed, Westwall.

Features: Native to North America, growing, depending on the plant, in several states and Canada, of which there are sixty in North America.

Though edible, starchy yet nutritious, the broad milky root is very bitter (the bitter outside slips off while boiling, as for food), and was an important food amongst Native Americans. Bitterroot is an evergreen, stem-less almost, with a rosette of oblong fleshy leaves. The flower emerges in the middle, is pink or white, and it normally stays open only in the sunlight from May to August.

Medicinal Part: Root.

Solvents: Alcohol, especially water.

Bodily Influence: Emetic, diaphoretic, tonic, laxative, expectorant.

Uses: Bitterroot is a popular cure for treating venereal diseases by Native Americans and is known as almost infallible. The management of Bright's disease has been recommended. It is also widely appreciated for rheumatic gout of the joints, and where anything else has collapsed, it has been known to alleviate cardiac dropsy. Parkinson cites it as a "sovereign cure against both poisons and sick dog bites"; it thus takes its name from dogbane. Bitterroot can help eliminate other impurities, including worms, from the bloodstream, and influence diabetes care. Bitterroot is a very bitter relaxing tonic that primarily works on the liver, empties the gall ducts, secures free bile waste, and thereby induces bowel movement. The bitterroot of the liver is unequalled with jaundice, gallstones, and chronic sluggish diseases. It should not be used for irritable stomach problems.

Dose: If used as an alternative to liver or dyspepsia, the dosage will be 10 grains twice a day, or 10 grains twice a day. Any nervous headache practitioners have employed this treatment, which is considered to be one of the most timely and effective treatments in use. Big amounts induce vomiting, but by incorporating peppermint (Mentha piperita), calamus (sweet flag), fennel (Foeniculum icinale), or other carminatives, the urge to grab may be removed. As a general tonic, take 2–5 grains thrice daily.

Note: Bitterroot milk can eliminate unsightly warts in the spring (if circulation is successful inside the system) if freshly added two to three times a day. Make sure to refer to the elevated area only. A burning and, perhaps, a swelling, you will notice; this is to be expected. If a scab forms the field, let it drop out on its own accord; a smooth, unelevated surface would be underneath. (Don't count moles as warts.)

2.4. BLACKBERRY - *Rubus Villosus*

Family: *Rosaceae*

Common Names: Dewberry, brambleberry, gout berry.

Features: There are various Rubus (blackberry) species; two types of trailing blackberries or dewberries and erect blackberries are known. There are, however, many intermediate types in both the wild and under cultivation. This unique variety is endemic to the northern United States and Canada, with central and Western Europe among other regions.

The blackberry has a root that lasts for several years and a top that grows with juicy, black, tasty berries one year and fruits the next. As for the regular raspberry, the berries stick to the heart when regular rather than withdrawing from the receptacle. When out of season, this trailing vine dies back on the field. In sandy or dry soil, spring finds clean, prickly tips that form rootlets. The blossoms are white.

Medicinal Parts: fruit, stems, leaves.

Solvents: Tobacco, water.

Influence Bodily: Astringent, tonic.

Uses: Blackberries are listed as astringent as a remedial agent and are much more medically serviceable than is understood to most of our generation. Native Americans used the berries as food and medication, and today we know from their history and clinical studies that the plant is highly useful for children's chronic diarrhoea, dysentery, cholera, and summer complaints and is sometimes the only thing that produces results.

Four or five times a day, a decoction of the root or leaves or both (the root being more astringent than the leaves) may be used openly. This agent is useful in prolonged menstruation and very productive in fevers and hot distempers of the body, ears, skin, and other parts, being pleasing to the mouth.

The berries can be turned into aspics, brandy, jam, jelly, as well as vinegar and have cordial properties.

Dose: one teaspoonful of root or leaves, steeped for 15 minutes to 1 cup of boiling water; 3-4 cups a day, depending on age and position. 1/2–1 dram of the tincture, three to four times a day.

Note: The swollen and outwardly rubbed leaves can serve as an astringent for haemorrhoids. Gargle the tea of the roots and leaves regularly for sore mouth and inflamed throat; they may be used green or dried.

Vintage illustration #5_Black Cohosh

2.5. BLACK COHOSH - *Cimicifuga Racemosa*

Family: *Ranunculaceae*

Common Names: Bugbane, rattle root, squawroot, snakeroot, black snakeroot.

Features: The plant is a genus of about twenty species in the crowfoot tribe, native to North America, Asia, and Europe.

Because of its medicinal properties, the best-known American species is the bugbane (Cimicifuga racemosa), Cimicifuga, so-called from the Latin "to hurry free," since certain species are used to expel bugs and other insects. It can also be used as an alternative to snake venom. In upland forests and hillsides, black cohosh can be used. An evergreen herb with a broad knotty root and a few small branches. With irregular leaves, the stem is plain, smooth, and furrowed, 3-9 feet long. In wand-like racemes, the small white flowers are widespread, flowering from May to August. There is a resin called cimicifugin (macrotin), sugar, gum, tannic acid, etc. in the root.

Part Medicinal: Root.

Solvent: Boiling water increases the root's properties but dissolves only partially; alcohol dissolves entirely.

Bodily Influence: alterative, diuretic, diaphoretic, expectorant, antispasmodic, cardiac stimulant (safer than digital), sedative (arterial and nervous), emmenagogue.

Uses: Native American women were conscious of black cohosh during the menstrual cycle for pain relief and widely used its products during childbirth.

In 1831, Dr. Young brought Cimicifuga racemosa to the field of medicine. Fatty heart, chorea, acute and chronic bronchitis, rheumatism, neuralgia, agitation, phthisis, dyspepsia, amenorrhea, dysmenorrhea, and seminal emission have been adapted as a cardiac tonic. Scarlet fever, pneumonia, and smallpox are all exemplary therapies. Considered by certain doctors to be one of the safest agents used for whooping cough.

- Two tablespoons of Black Cohosh Tincture (Cimicifuga racemosa)
- Two spoons of bloodroot tincture (Sanguinaria canadensis)

- Two teaspoons of lobelia (Lobelia inflata) tincture
- Two tablespoons of Squill Syrup (sea onion)

Dose: Every three to four hours, 15 to 30 drops

In Saint Vitus's dance and in asthma, delirium tremens, consumption, acute rheumatism, scrofula, and leukorrhea, the above tinctures have been successfully used. Big doses are responsible for vertigo, tremors, heartbeat drop, dehydration, and prostration.

Caution: Pregnant women do not use this medication.

Dose: The tincture should be produced from fresh root or from a recently dried root; 2 ounces to 2 ounces of the tincture.

1. 5 to 15 drops four times a day, 1/2 pint of alcohol (96 proof) taken.
2. Three times a day, or 15 to 30 drops of tincture applied to 1 cup of sugar, sweetened with butter, as a drink, one teaspoonful of the cut root to 1 cup of boiling water.

Note: The wounded root was used as a snakebite remedy, added to the wound by the Native Americans, and the juice was administered internally in very small quantities.

2.6. BLACK ROOT - *Veronicastrum Virgin Icum*

Family: *Plantaginaceae*

Common Names: Culver's physic, tall speedwell, leptandra, Culver's root.

Features: The black root comes from the figwort genus, which is endemic to North America.

The soil where the plant is grown has a major impact on its virtues. In fresh soils, damp forests, swamps, etc., it can be observed. The medicinal benefit is improved by Limestone soil, guaranteeing the consumer of its attributed impact.

The correct time for the meeting is the fall of the second year. The most agreed procedure is dried root (fresh root is too irritable), but it must be used with great caution.

With simple, straight, smooth, herbaceous roots, the plant reaches heights of 2 to 5 feet. The leaves, whorled into fours to sevens, are low and finely serrated. The flowers are white, almost sessile, and they are very numerous.

Calyx: corolla with four sections, small and almost white. The Stamens: two. The fruit is a capsule containing several seeds.

Taste: Acrid, very bitter.

Medicinal Part: root dried.

Solvents: Tobacco, water.

Bodily Influence: Emetocathartic, alterative, tonic, antiseptic.

Uses: A long-established Native American remedy is black root. It was invented as a therapeutic agent by Dr. Culver as a white man's medication and is beautifully referred to as Culver's physics.

The black root's key importance is that when there is inadequate biliary flow, it works on the intestines in chronic constipation and is quite commonly used in chronic hepatic diseases. As is so common with other purgative drugs, it acts moderately and without depressing the brain.

It eliminates the gruesome matter from the intestines in fevers without reducing their tone or leaving behind the dangerous sting that remains even after calomel is used. It is very successfully used in the treatment of pleurisy and also in certain cases of dyspepsia. As dysentery cathartic, when given in moderate doses, it is one of the best medicines available. Combine with a small rhubarb root (Rheum palmatum) in such situations and give the decoction in doses of 3-4 teaspoons, repeating until passively satisfied every three hours.

In this, you have a superior herbal remedy to most traditional treatments and one that has been used for centuries.

Dose: Leptandrin is a root extract; it can be used in smaller quantities, from 1/4 to 1 grain, balanced by age and situation. A dosage of 20-40 grains of sand, like a cathartic.

For Liver Diseases Formula:

- 1 ounce (Veronicastrum virginicum) black root
- Goldenseal 2 ounces (Hydrastis canadensis)
- 2 ounces (Cassia marilandica) of senna
- Two pints of water that is bottled or boiled.
- Boil until it has decreased to 1 pint.
- Three to four times a day, take two teaspoons, raising the volume if it fails to operate softly to lowering if it works too much.

2.7. BLACK WALNUT - *Juglans Nigra*

Family: *Walnut*

Features: Six species of walnuts, the Juglans family, derived from the United States. Among them is black walnut, generally spread in the eastern states and spreading to neighbouring Canada. Rough furrowed bark, alternating pinnately clustered leaves with a distinctive odour when battered, and greenish flowers, the male in drooping catkins, are these deciduous hardwoods.

One of the best-known, largest, and most important native hardwoods is the black walnut. While not widespread, the tree grows rapidly on thick, wet, well-drained soil in mixed forests, as is found in valleys. It reaches 100 feet in height occasionally, with trunks 3 feet in diameter. Planted as ornamentals for roadside shade and shelterbelts.

The wood is beautifully crafted and used as panelling, for building furniture, and in salad bowls.

Nuts are a common food for flavouring sweets, ice cream, and cake. Like the hickory nut, the husk does not break open; when on the tree, it is coated with a green pulp covering that becomes black while on the ground and in storage. For dyeing and tanning, this external pulp is used. You will remember the leftover walnut stains, whether you have ever collected or hulled black walnuts.

Parts of Medicinal: bark, berries, rind, green nuts.

Solvents: Water, marijuana.

Bodily Influence: Tonic, Vermifuge.

Uses: Materially, with one cup of the leaves boiling in 1 quart of water, made fresh every day and sometimes used with honey, the scrofula had harmonious results. For several months, this should be continued. When the green may not be had, the dry leaves can be used. In bilious and cramp colic treatment, a good tincture of the leaves and nuts is extremely exalted as an antidote.

Dose: Every twenty to thirty minutes, 1-2 teaspoonfuls until relieved. It is also successful to use a decoction as a vermifuge. In diphtheria, the rind of the green fruit extracts the ringworm and tetter and is given. The fermented fresh walnuts relax hysteria, core, and pregnant vomiting in spirit alcohol.

One of the foods high in manganese, vital for nerves, brain, and cartilage, is the black walnut.

The Missouri black walnut is nutritionally rich in manganese. Both nut fruits, as rancid oil is counterproductive, should be young.

One teaspoonful of inner bark or leaves and rind, sliced into 1 cup of boiling water, thin or granulated.

Drink 1-4 cups a day, a huge mouthful at a time, always.

2.8. BLOODROOT - *Sanguinaria Canadensis*

Family: *Papaveraceae*

Common Names: Red puccoon, Indian plant, tetterwort, sanguinaria.

Features: Bloodroot, a monotypic genus of the Papaveraceae family, is endemic to eastern North America.

In its forest habitat, where sheltered areas and leaf mould are suitable for its survival, the tiny herb is always hard to locate. The dense, palmately lobed leaf is lapped around the bud, which rapidly outgrows its guardian, drops its two brief sepals, and opens into a star-shaped bloom, one on each stem, within its middle many fleshy white petals and a mass of gold stamens.

The flower shuts at night or on shady days and is among the flowers in the early spring. It is also grown in gardens. During the summer, the leaves begin to grow, being almost 7 inches long. The seeds are found in capsules that are spindle shaped.

The entire plant is very brittle and succulent, and an acrid red juice bleeds from the divided parts when damaged, particularly at its thick, fleshy root. The root is approximately the size of the little finger of a guy. The flavour is rough and salty. The entire plant is medicinal, the root being mostly the component used. The structures are affected by age and moisture.

Part Medicinal: Root.

Solvent: Water, alcohol.

Bodily Influence: systemic emetic, expectorant stimulator, sialagogue, alterative, tonic, febrifuge, diuretic.

Uses: Used by the colonists for all blood conditions and as a dye on their skin and as a cosmetic colorant. Bloodroot behaviour varies according to management. It activates the digestive organs in small amounts and serves as a stimulant and tonic; it is an arterial sedative in high doses. In chronic bronchitis, laryngitis, croup, pneumonia, whooping cough, and other respiratory organ problems, the symptoms are beneficial. The tincture has been used effectively in chest dyspepsia and dropsy, and in cases of catarrh or bloated, morbid, or jaundiced liver disorders. The operation of this large glandular organ, whose proper function is so essential for our daily lives' full physical and mental makeup, is triggered by Bloodroot.

Caution: Usage as instructed only. Big amounts are lethal.

Dose: one stage of a teaspoonful of grated root steeped for half an hour in 1 pint of boiling water. Cold, strain, take three to six times a day for a teaspoonful. Ice as an emetic, 10-20 grains; stimulant and expectorant ice, 3-5 grains; alternate powder, 1/2-2 grains. 20–60 drops of tincture.

Note: injections of solid tea are excellent for leukorrhea and haemorrhoids. As an external treatment, in cases of fungal tumours, ringworm, tetter, warts, etc., the powdered root or tincture works vigorously at the same time as stated, to be taken internally. A snuff of ground bloodroot is also used to treat the nasal polypus.

2.9. BEARBERRY - *Uva Ursi*

Family: *Ericaceae*

Common Names: Arberry, Arbousier, Arbousier Traînant, Arbutus uva-ursi, Arctostaphylos uva-ursi

Features: Uva ursi is a shrub that grows flowers and berries. The leaves are used to make medicine.

Bears are particularly fond of uva ursi berries. This explains the Latin name, "uva ursi," which means "bear's grape." Most authorities refer to Arctostaphylos uva-ursi as uva ursi. Do not confuse this plant with Arctostaphylos adentricha and Arctostaphylos coactylis, which have also been referred to as uva ursi.

Uses: Uva ursi is used for infections of the kidney, bladder, or urethra (urinary tract infections or UTIs) and swelling (inflammation) of the urinary tract, but there is no good scientific evidence to support these uses. Research shows that taking uva ursi for 3-5 days does not improve symptoms of a UTI or reduce the need for antibiotics.

Uva ursi can reduce bacteria in the urine. It can also reduce swelling (inflammation) and have a drying (astringent) effect on the tissues.

More evidence is needed to rate the effectiveness of uva ursi for these uses: Constipation, kidney infections, bronchitis.

Dose: When taken by mouth: Uva ursi is possibly safe for most adults when taken for up to one month. It can cause nausea, vomiting, stomach discomfort, and a greenish-brown discoloration of the urine.

The appropriate dose of uva ursi depends on several factors such as the user's age, health, and several other conditions. At this time there is not enough scientific information to determine an appropriate range of doses for uva ursi. Keep in mind that natural products are not always necessarily safe and dosages can be important. Be sure to follow relevant directions on product labels and consult your pharmacist or physician or other healthcare professional before using.

Caution: Uva ursi is possibly unsafe when taken in high doses for more than one month. It can cause liver damage, breathing problems, convulsions, and death when used in high doses. When used for a long time, it might increase the risk for cancer.

- Pregnancy and breast-feeding: Using uva ursi during pregnancy is likely unsafe because it might start labor. There isn't enough reliable information to know if uva ursi is safe to use when breast-feeding. Stay on the safe side and avoid use.

- Children: Uva ursi is possibly unsafe in children when taken by mouth. Uva ursi contains a chemical that might cause severe liver problems. Do not give uva ursi to children.

- Retinal thinning: Uva ursi contains a chemical that can thin the retina in the eye. This could worsen the condition of people whose retinas are already too thin. Avoid use if you have this problem.

- Be cautious with this combination: lithium interacts with Uva ursi.

- Uva ursi might have an effect like a water pill or "diuretic." Taking uva ursi might decrease how well the body gets rid of lithium. This could increase how much lithium is in the body and result in serious side effects. Talk with your healthcare provider before using this product if you are taking lithium. Your lithium dose might need to be changed.

2.10. CAPSICUM - *Capsicum Minimum, C. Frutescens*

Family: *Solanaceae*

Common Names: Cayenne, red pepper, bird pepper, African pepper.

Features: Along the southern line of Tennessee, this plant is endemic to portions of the United States, Asia and Africa. The African bird pepper is technically the purest and the best known. It is a small, oblong, scarlet, membranous pod that is internally divided into two or three cells containing various smooth, white, reniform seeds. It has no smell; it has a hot and acrid flavour.

Solvents: 98% alcohol, vinegar to a large degree, boiling water.

Part Medicinal: Fruit

Bodily Influence: Stimulant, tonic, carminative, diaphoretic, rubefacient, condiment

Uses: The capsicum calming effect is the root of its internal efficacy. Capsicum taken with burdock, goldenseal, ginger, slippery elm, etc., will quickly disperse through the whole system, equalizing circulation in all diseases caused by circulation obstruction. Unlike other allopathy stimulants, it is not a narcotic medication.

It primarily works on the blood, providing an acute effect on the heart and then spreading to the capillaries, without increasing the rhythm, toning the bloodstream.

Note that it is an agent rarely used alone, and it is quickly extinguished by itself. Cayenne is effective for coughs, kidney torpor, diarrhoea, pleurisy, typhoid fever, stomach, and intestinal cramps and pains, triggering the previously contracted sections' prolonged movement. With Dr. R. Swinburne Clymer named it "the only natural stimulant worth trying with muddy mucus stools and aggressive breath in diarrhoea and dysentery." Lung bleeding is quickly tested through the use of cayenne and a vapor wash. Circulation is facilitated across the body by this process, decreasing pressure on the lungs and thereby providing a chance for a coagulum to develop around ruptured vessels. When followed by a cup of hot herb tea, the uncomfortable sensation of indigestion or heartburn suffered by several individuals when taking cayenne capsules or tablets will vanish. The cause of the unpleasantness is normally not Cayenne. With all its positive capacity, the Constitution fights against disease and bad emotions, and it is by this force of re-action that disease is defeated. Capsicum is not a cure-all, and given the findings available, we do not advocate its continuous use (except for cooking).

Note: For the treatment of sprains, fractures, rheumatism, and neuralgia:

- Tincture of capsicum, 2 ounces of blood
- Fluid lobelia extract (Lobelia inflata), 2 fluid ounces.
- Wormwood Oil (Artemisia obsinthiura)
- Rosemary Oil, 1 Fluidram
- Spear Gasoline, 1 Fluidram

According to the Back to Eden review, by J. Kloss, capsicum contains albumin, pectin, strange gum, starch, lime carbonate, iron sesquioxide, potash phosphate, alum, magnesia, and oil of a reddish nature.

Vintage illustration #7_Capsicum

2.11. CATNIP - *Nepeta Cataria*

Family: *Lamiaceae*

Common names: Catnip, nep, Catmint, Wort of the Cat.

Features: All parts of the United States contain this naturalized perennial plant. Fine whitish hairs cover the circular, straight, branching stems; leaves 1-2 1/2 inches long with heart-shaped or oblong spiked top, the upper side green with underlying greyish green and whitish hairs. In-flowering
With whitish corolla, purple-dotted, sectioned cheeks, and lobes defining the bloom conformation, June to September. The scent is mildly minty, with a sour flavour.

Solvents: Hot water, dissolved spirits.

Medicinal Part: The herb in its entirety.

Bodily Influence: Carminative, stimulant, tonic, diaphoretic, emmenagogue, antispasmodic, aphrodisiac (cats).

Uses: Sadly, when most of us hear of catnip, we just equate it with the cat's kin. The applications for both infants and adults are numerous and mild in the right concentrations. The American physio-medical profession advises "blood warm bowel infusion injection for infants with intestinal flatulence" when disturbed by flatulence and digestive pains. Both herbalists deem catnip helpful for feverish colds. Without increasing the temperature, it will create perspiration and cause sleep. It has been shown to be effective in alleviating acute nervous headache and anxiety, paranoia, and other types of nervous disorders, without any withdrawal effect when withdrawn.

In scarlet fever, smallpox, colds, etc., equivalent sections of catnip and saffron are exceptional. It will stimulate suppressed menstruation by the fresh articulated juice of the green herb taken in tablespoonful amounts three times a day. Because of its temporary operation, in tea form, catnip is more serviceable. In a closed jar, still steep the plant, never simmer.

Dose: 1 ounce of boiling water per 1 pint of catnip. Adults, 2-3 tablespoons; youth, 2-3 teaspoons, mostly, for the above. It frequently causes emesis if taken in very large doses when warm.

Note: Culpeper states that the bruised green herb applied to the rectum for 2-3 hours relieves haemorrhoid pain. For the same purpose, the juice that is made into an ointment is effective. There is an old saying that it would make the calmest person fierce and quarrelsome if the root is chewed.

2.12. CHAMOMILE - *Chamaemelum Nobile*

Family: *Asteraceae*

Common Names: German chamomile, chamomile from the garden, field fruit, pinheads.

Features: The beloved chamomile originates in southern Europe and is legally referred to as Anthemis
Nobilis (Roman chamomile), with superior medicinal properties to ours.
This thin, daisy-like perennial, yellow or whitish, with a strong fibrous root and pale green, thread-shaped leaflet.

Taste: It has a very bitter flavour, with a strong aromatic apple odour. It is important to notice that chamomile, meaning "land apple," is derived from the Greek name.

Medicinal Parts: Medicinal flowers.

Solvents: Tobacco, water.

Bodily Influence: Stomachic, antispasmodic, carminative, diaphoretic, tonic stimulant (volatile oil), nervine, sedative, emmenagogue.

Uses: Chamomile is one of the herbs that are well known. Its livelihood may be developed by its early use in childhood diseases such as colds, infantile seizures, stomach pain, colic, earache, restlessness, measles, etc. If kids were treated with chamomile now, we may have less of the chronic diseases that bother us in later years.

When wet, chamomile stimulates perspiration and softens the skin. During convalescence from febrile illness, dyspepsia, both triggers of the weak or irritable stomach, persistent and typhoid fever, the cold injection serves as a tonic and is most fitting for stomach disorders, and as a cocktail. According to age, take 2-3 teaspoons, or a cupful, changed two or three times a day.

Using white flowers (fresh or dried) with strong white wine, a syrup made from chamomile juice is a tonic for jaundice and drops. Old-fashioned but worth recalling in women for emotional and anxious affections can stimulate menstrual discharge, alleviate dysmenorrhoeal spasms, and facilitate menstruation when exposure to colds is delayed, for uterine spasms or anxious stress, bilious headache, and digestive help. Specific to the mother's uterus pain during nursing.

Note: The chamomile flower, pounded and turned into oil, comforts the agony of the liver and spleen; drink fresh or dried herb tea at the same time. Culpeper states: "A stone taken out of the human body, wrapped in Chamomile, will melt in time, and a little too."

When all ways have fallen, the flowers combined with crushed poppy head make a good poultice for allaying pains. It is also excellent as a lotion for outward use in toothaches, earaches, neuralgia, etc.

A chamomile poultice also stops and eliminates gangrene while present. For sprains and fractures, the battered and vinegar-moistened herb is great. For soapwort, it can be rendered up

(Saponaria) into a shampoo, especially to keep fair hair alive and healthy.

2.13. CENTAURY - *Centaurium Erytraea*

Family: *Gentianaceae*

Common names: pink rose, sour clover, sour bloom.

Features: This plant is common and endemic in most parts of the U.S. There are numerous organisms and colours; by using the red centaury in blood diseases, the yellow in choleric diseases, and the white in those in phlegm and water, the English differentiate between them. Variety is not limited to colour only; in many soil environments, the centaury family can grow wet meadows, high grass, prairies, and damp ditch soil. From June to September, it flowers and is better harvested at this time. At night, the flowers close, and the American variety is known to be superior to the European one.

Solvents: Tobacco, water.

Medicinal part: The herb in its entirety.

Bodily influence: Tonic, febrifuge, diaphoretic:

Uses: Great old American antidote, bitter tonic, prevention against all periodic febrile disorders, dyspepsia and fever convalescence, tightening the stomach, and encouraging digestion. Help for both joint pains and rheumatic pains. The following is a domestic treatment for expelling worms and recovering menstrual secretions in a warm infusion: of the powder, 1/2-1 dram; of the extract, 2-6 grams. One teaspoonful to 1 cup of boiling water, a loose dried leaf. This powerful plant, while bitter, is a pleasant accompaniment to all herbal teas and preparations. Mix with other herbs for taste, such as anise, cardamom, peppermint, ginger, fennel, etc.

Vintage illustration #8_Centuary

2.14. CHAGA - *Inonotus Obliquus*

Family: *Hymenochaetaceae*

Common names: Chaga, birch mushroom.

Features: In North America and Canada, the birch is recognized only for its elegance. A mushroom, or fungus-type formation, occurring in older trees (also growing on beech and other trees), serves its medical function. Often hold Chaga in a dry and dark position (dark covered jar) as its strength is dissipated by dampness and bright light.

Medicinal part: The granular portions of the three layers within.

Solvents: Water that is heated (not heated), tobacco, whisky.

Bodily influence: tonic, purifying semen, anodyne, restorative.

Uses: It is well known that all plants and how they were best used for fruit, medicine, even whether they were poisonous, were known to the Native Americans. We recognize in Anglo-American literature that therapies of certain illnesses have been preserved as tribal information. We recognize that they have used many fungi properties, but we cannot locate a definitive record of Chaga being described from our laboratory work; we are poorly educated.

2.15. CHERRY - *Prunus Virginiana*

Family: *Rosaceae*

Common names: Chokecherry, wild black cherry.

Features: Native to North America, this massive fruit tree is found in Canada, Florida, Minnesota, Nebraska, Kansas, Louisiana, and Texas.

The bark on the outside is blackish and rough. The young branches are glossy, red or purple; in May and June, flowers emerge after the leaves, followed in August by a delicious cherry. When macerated in water, the bark has a strong aromatic scent that resembles bitter almond; the taste is astringent and slightly bitter. The fresh, thin bark is the best; there should be rejection of very large or small branches. Stem bark is gathered and thoroughly dried in the autumn; sloughing dead tissue should be discarded if present.

In a closed container in a dark spot, it will survive well.

Solvent: Vapor that's hot or cold.

Medicinal part: Thin young bark.

Bodily influence: Mild tonic, calming astringent, sedative, pectoral.

Uses: As a vehicle base, wild cherry bark is commonly used in cough medicines. In many other disease types, this agent is useful. It is outstanding in the form of syrup for children's diarrhoea, which can be pleasantly combined with cordial neutralization; indigestion caused by a loss of stomach tone can be greatly relieved. Relieves asthma, bronchitis, scrofula, palpitation of the heart (not to be seen with dry cough), dyspepsia, hectic fever, deterioration in chronic and damaged cases in throat and chest coughing. A small amount of hydrocyanic acid is found in it. The cherry is rich in life-giving properties and contains malic acid.

Homeopathic Clinical: Cold injection or inner bark tincture; solution of distilled resin extract, acidity pruning, anorexia, dyspepsia, cardiac, pyrosis.

Dose: Fifteen drops of vapor. Cherry bark will remove kidney and bladder stones, but it should be mixed and cautiously treated with other herbs over a span of several months; the stones will be removed without softening when extracted too soon.

2.16. CHESTNUT - *Castanea Dentata*

Introduced herb.

Family: *Fagaceae*

Common Names: American chestnut, Spanish chestnut, sweet chestnut.

Features: In North America, western Asia, and southern Europe, this stately chestnut tree grows. Typically, the plant is self-sterile, requiring more than one tree for chestnut output. The flowers consist of long catkins that can contain or be solely male or female, or fruit-bearing, organs at their base. They grow spiny burrs containing 1-5 single-seeded nuts if the female flowers are fertilized. Overhead, the leaves are dark green, light below, partially torn, twisted, or matted, with a light odor and an astringent flavour. Chestnuts are low in calcium, heavy in starch and carbohydrates, and contain minerals such as potash phosphate, magnesia, calcium, and titanium.

Medicinal Parts: Inner bark, leaves.

Solvents: boiling water (partial solvent) alcohol.

Bodily influence: Mild sedative, astringent, tonic.

Use: Culpeper said the inner skin containing the nut "is of such a binding nature that a scruple taken by a man or ten grains by a boy easily prevents any flux at all." It is believed to be specific for whooping cough or nagging distressing coughs, paroxysm management, and for recurrent hiccups and other irritable and excitable symptoms of the pulmonary organs. The green or dried leaves should be used. Fevers respond to the relaxing of the mucous surfaces and the nervous system, acting as an antispasmodic agent. The most effective mixture of the above is Lobelia inflata and Caulophyllum thalictroides (blue cohosh).

Dose: 1 ounce to 1 pint of boiling water with a 15-minute infusion. A wineglass three times a day, half the number for girls. It is safe to use the fluid extract: dosage 10 drops three times a day; 5 drops for girls.

Caution: The introduced blight has caused substantial damage to Castanea dentata in recent years. Do not use the horse chestnut (Aesculus hippocastanum), which is now more widely encountered and has a bitter and slightly poisonous fruit.

2.17. CHICKWEED - *Stellaria Media*

Family: *Caryophyllaceae*

Common Names: Stitchwort, flower of satin mouth of adder, starweed.

Features: On the American continent, there are around twenty-five native and naturalized species. For several years, Native Americans used native chickweed but sometimes introduced naturalized plants. It is widespread in Europe and America, growing in damp, shady areas in fields and around dwellings. The stem is thin and straggling, widely branched; there is only a line of white hair on one side, with each pair of leaves shifting direction. From the beginning of spring before fall, the very tiny white flowers bloom. It tastes a bit salty. Poultry and birds ingest the plants.

Solvents: Tobacco, water.

Medicinal part: Whole medicines.

Bodily influence: Demulcent, emollient, pectoral, coolant.

Uses: This so-called nuisance garden weed soothes and cures multiple regions of internal inflammation. There are many applications, from salad greens to poultices, ads, and raw, dry, or powdered herb salves. This plant is used to alleviate haemorrhoids, for liver diseases (internally and externally), bronchitis, pleurisy, cough, colds, hoarseness, rheumatism, infection or weakening of the intestines and throat, lungs, bronchial tubes, scurvy, kidney disorders, to open the tiny arteries that carry blood from the liver through the hepatic veins, making them more pliable. Among the all-purpose herbals, this so-called popular plant could be included.

Dose: 1 chickweed ounce per 1 1/2 pints of water, simmered down to 1 pint, per 2-3 hours, a wineglassful. For inflamed surfaces, boils, and skin eruptions, apply externally as a poultice.

Note: Beneficial with any swelling, facial redness, weakening, scabs, boiling, burning, swollen or sore eyes, erysipelas, cancers, haemorrhoids, cancer-swollen testicles, ulcerated throat, and lips. It is an efficient medication for fractured or unbroken skin disorders.

Vintage illustration #11_Chickweed

2.18. DAMIANA - *Turnera Dif Usa Var. Aphrodisiaca*

Family: *Turneraceae*

Features: Indigenous to Texas, California, and South America. There are long, large, obovate, light green leaves in the small yellow-flowered shrub, a few hairs on the ribs, along with reddish twigs. The plant has an aromatic fragrance and contains volatile oil with a wet, bitter, camphor-like flavour (0.51 percent), two resins, a bitter concept (Damiani), tannin, sugar, and albuminoids.

Part medicinal: Leaves.

Solvent: Alcohol with dilution.

Bodily influence: Aphrodisiac, tonic, laxative, stimulant.

Uses: As a major sexual rejuvenator of sexual organ lethargy, whether the product of trauma or senility, Damiana has clear arguments. The usage, or management, should be careful since those who know of its power explain the statements. For anyone who can need it, please note that damiana frequently activates beyond the limits of protection and health when the device is worn down, overworked, subjected to nervous pressures, etc.; stimulation above our normal energy level may have a detrimental impact on the heart.

There are several objections to its effect on the digestive tract, but this risk is partially dismissed in combination with phosphorus and nux vomica. The intensity required would not necessarily be known. Usually, one section once a day for ten days. It is also used for nervous disorders.

Dose: Fluid extract, once a day, 15-30 drops. 3–6 grains, strong extract. Used in pill shape as well.

2.19. DANDELION - *Taraxacum Of Icinale*

Family: *Asteraceae*

Common names: Blast ball, cankerwort, lion's teeth, wild endive, etc.

Features: This plant is endemic to Greece but can now be found nearly all year round in most parts of the world. Taraxacum is a genus belonging to the sunflower family (Compositae) of fewer than one hundred species of biennial or perennial plants.

Dandelions are distinguished by glossy green leaf rosettes, in a marginally backward direction, almost entirely or variously tooth edged. The flower base, bearing a single yellow flower, is longer than the leaves, 5-6 inches in height. When sliced, the root and stem yield a milky substance. When the plant is in the fall, the root is the official component that should be gathered.

In salads, spring leaves are used and have some mild narcotic properties. In bloom from April to November, it can be seen outside most doors across the United States. Dry some of your once thought-of-as-worthless winter dandelion roots, which will benefit you in several ways.

Part medicinal: Root.

Solvents: Water to simmer, marijuana.

Bodily influence: Diuretic, tonic, stomachic, perennial. The great importance of the dandelion was known by Native Americans and used as food and medicine.

Uses: The common dandelion was intelligently used as a medicinal plant. It contains 7,000 units of vitamin A per ounce and is an outstanding source of vitamins B, C, and G. For contrast, the content of vitamin A in lettuce is 1,200 units per ounce and 1,275 units per ounce in carrots. A wise and simple contribution to our food.

It has an opening and cleaning quality and is also useful for liver, gallbladder, and spleen obstructions and diseases originating from the biliary organs. It is a great agent for skin infections, scurvy, eczema, and scrofula; it has a positive effect on the female organs. Dandelion is used more commonly by herbalists than any other herb, as it blends well with other liver herbal preparations and is mild, wholesome, and healthy. For all rheumatic complaints, its extended application may only be helpful. Twenty-eight parts of sodium are the normal dietary salt in dandelion; this organic sodium source purifies the blood and removes the acids therein.

Eden Kloss tells us: *"Anemia is caused by the absence of dietary salts in the blood, which actually has little to do with the consistency of healthy blood."* Dandelion root is sliced, which is dried up by health-minded people for coffee. From a wellness standpoint, consuming is more desirable than coffee or tea. It is sometimes mixed with roasted acorns and roasted rye in equal parts, or according to taste, for this reason. It is unmatched as a vegetable for salads, being abundant in many minerals. It's a farm with medicinal vegetables.

It is known that the roots were used as a sedative as early as the sixteenth century in Germany.

Dose: 5–40 drops of the tincture. Fill a cup with the green leaves for infusions, apply hot water, steep water, and 1/2 or more hours. Drink three or four times a day when you are cold. Or in 1 cup of boiling water, add one teaspoon of cut or ground root and steep for 1/2 hour. Drink three times a day when you are cold.

Uses: The root is the most common in Russia, prepared as an extract with vodka, tea, or coffee. Ancient home medicine names it "existence elixir," and it is known as an expectorant and sedative for the purification of blood, liver care, jaundice, gallbladder, skin disorders, and digestive disorder. Clinically: in the form of oils, tinctures, powders, loose and in tablets, for the above conditions which have been long known.

2.20. ECHINACEA - *Echinacea Angustifolia*

Family: *Asteraceae*

Common names: Purple coneflower, black Sampson.

Features: Native to America's prairie regions west of Ohio. The aster family belongs to this native herbaceous perennial. With short, stout, bristly, hairy roots, the plant grows 2–3 feet long. Leaves are compact, rough, rugged, narrowly landscaped, narrower at the top, 3-8 inches long. From July to October, the single, large flower head emerges, the colour ranging from whitish rose to deep purple. The taste is sweetish, then tingling, as in aconite, except when improperly administered without its continuous benumbing effect. Faint odour, fragrant, and should not be used after the signature odour and flavour have been lost. It includes tissue of inulin-bearing parenchyma.

Medicinal parts: root, dried rhizome.

Solvent: Beer.

Bodily influence: Sialagogue, diaphoretic, alterative.

Uses: Useful for all infections caused by blood impurities. Echinacea is a natural herbal antitoxin, Thompsonian, and physio-medical practitioners and naturopaths have often maintained.

Orthodox doctors, though many have, have not traditionally been able to recognize it as such. While disagreement is allowed, misinformation is more fake, and reality is truer.

Echinacea is a corrector of fluid body deprivations, as Dr. Niederkorn noticed, and this is because the morbid shifts in body fluids are internal or caused by external introductions.

Echinacea is known for septic diseases, septicemia in its multiple ways, blood poisoning, dynamic fever, typhoid fever, cellular abscesses, salpingitis, carbohydrates, cancerous cachexia, and for fevers or disorders in which the mucous membranes are bullishly discolored; for any sepsis-pointing disease, internal or external.

For hydrophobia, snakebite, and septicemia, the Sioux tribe used fresh scraped roots.

Dose: Steep one teaspoonful of the granulated root in one cup of boiling water for 1/2-hour, strain, three to six times daily for one tablespoonful. 5-10 min. of the tincture.

Note: Steep as above and remove the sections involved or bathe them.

2.21. ELDER - *Sambucus Canadensis*

Family: *Adoxaceae*

Common names: Sambucus, American elder, sweet elder.

Features: An exotic shrub native to America. It is found poor, moist lands, thickets, and waste places in all areas of the United States and Canada. For their ornamental foliage, the elders are also cultivated. With star-shaped, fragrant flowers 1/4-inch-wide, arranged in flat flower clusters about 8 inches wide, they rise 5-12 feet high, blooming in June and July. In September and October, purple-black berries that produce three or four round seeds mature. Sometimes, the fruit is made into jellies, desserts, and wine. A rough, pitted grey bark covers the branching stems; large central stems are smooth. The fragrance is mildly sweet and floral. Taste: sour mildly. The European elder is comparable in general features and properties, but bigger than the American.

Medicinal parts: As a natural medicinal remedy, the roots, inner bark, plants, berries, and flowers are all known.

Solvent: With water.

Bodily influence: Emetic, Cathartic, Hydragogue. Flowers: diaphoretic, diuretic, alterative, emollient, debatable, stimulant gentle.

Uses: In circumstances of headache attributable to colds, palsy, rheumatism, scrofula, syphilis, jaundice, kidney disorders, and epilepsy, the fruits, fruit, herbs, inner bark, and roots have elicited appreciation from several.

Dr. Brown (1875) gives us the following: "Hydragogue, emetic, and cathartic is the Elder's inner bark."

By taking it from trees 1 or 2 years old, scraping off the grey outer bark, and steeping 2 ounces of it in 5 ounces of boiling water for 48 hours, it has been effectively used in epilepsy. Strain to send the patient a wineglass every 15 minutes if the fit is challenging. Resume it every 6 to 8 days. The flowers' tea is quieting, taken internally, despite twitching and irritation of the skin. Over closed lids, the tea simmered for 10 minutes longer, and cotton immersed in the solution gives an eye treatment. Therefore, the berries are rich in organic iron and are an excellent addition, especially if anaemic, to the autumn menu.

Combine 1 ounce of elderberry juice and blackberry juice three times a day.

The inner green bark is cathartic; its infusion into wine or conveyed juice is mildly purified in doses of 1/2 to 1 fluid ounce. Vomiting generates a significant dosage. It creates an efficient obstruent in small doses, facilitating all the fluid secretion, which is used a lot in dropsy to remove the water from the engorged body. Any other drug hardly overshadows it. It may be used for childhood disorders, such as liver abnormalities, erysipelas, etc., varying the volume by age.

Note: The elder can be called the cosmetic tree of the herbalist, as each component can assist in the beauty of the body, removing wrinkles, relieving inflammation, eliminating freckles, and maintaining and softening the skin if diligently, internally and externally applied.

2.22. FEVERFEW - *Chrysanthemum Parthenium*

Introduced herb.

Family: *Asteraceae*

Common names: Feather few, febrifuge plant, feather foil, pyrethrum.

Features: The plant is native to Europe but widespread in the U.S. Occasionally found in a wild state, but usually grown in gardens. A significant proportion of inulin is contained by the tapering base, with dark brown, furrowed bark. The yellowish, porous wood, with its sialagogue influence, has a distinct odour and a sweetish taste, very pungent, acrid, and tingling.

The herb is like chamomile with a yellow disc and white stalk-like petals, flowering in June and July. With serrated-edge alternate leaves, the middle stem grows to about 2 feet high; the hairs are very small.

Bees are reported to hate this plant very much, and they will be led to keep their distance by a handful of flower heads borne in their vicinity.

Medicinal part: The herb in its entirety.

Solvents: alcohol (partial solvent) hot water.

Bodily influence: Aperient, carminative, tonic, emmenagogue, vermifuge, stimulant

Uses: Feverfew's warming injection activates the skin, nervous system, and genitourinary organs and relieves dizziness, brain and nerve pressure, and overexcitation pressures in the head. When administered too liberally, Culpeper advises it as *"a peculiar cure against morphine."*

In cases of colic, flatulence, general indigestion, colds, suppressed urine, expelling larvae, vomiting, and in certain febrile diseases, this garden herb offers relieving assistance from hyperaemic disorders of the mucous membrane.

In female correction of scanty or irregular monthly cycles, it is largely used.

Dose: Dr. Clymer, interacting with the curing agents of nature, administers fevers as follows:

- Feverfew (Chrysanthemum parthenium) tincture, 10–30 drops
- Coneflower (Echinacea Angustifolia) tincture, 10-20 drops
- Cayenne pepper tincture, 10–20 drops

The dose of feverfew alone: 10-30 drops every 2-3 hours in the water. One teaspoonful to one cup of boiling water steeped for 1/2 hour should be used as a tea: two cups a day in small mouthful amounts.

Note: Hot compressed leaves are helpful for the discomfort of congestion or inflammation of the lungs, stomach, and abdomen.

2.23. GRAVEL ROOT - *Eutrochium Purpureum*

Family: *daisy*

Common Names: Eupatoire Pourpre, Herbe de Joe Pye, Eupatorium purpureum

Medicinal Part: The root, bulb, and above the ground growing parts are used in making medicine.

Uses: People use this for disorders such as urinary infections, pain in arthritis, fever, kidney stones, and many others, despite safety issues, but there's no good clinical proof to endorse these applications.

For some circumstances, the gravel root can function by minimizing swelling (inflammation).

With gravel root, lithium interacts well.

Inducers of Cytochrome P450 3A4 improve the breakdown of other drugs by the liver associate with gravel root.

Dose: The acceptable gravel root dosage depends on many variables, such as the age, fitness, and many other factors of the user. There is not adequate clinical evidence currently available to establish the optimal doses range for gravel root.

2.24. HOPS - *Humulus Lupulus*

Family: *Cannabaceae*

Features: The hop plant is a long-lived perennial dioecious propagated from rhizome sections or 'core cuttings' commercially. The hop is one of the few plant species of which various plants bear male and female flowers. The cones and stro-biles, which are used medicinally and in the processing of beer, ale, and porter, were introduced and grown in the United States.The stem is hard, very long, and any neighbouring reinforcement will curl around. Pairs of stems stalked, serrated, cordate. Yellowish green, oval, reticulate, veined, almost 1⁄2-inch-long are three- or five-lobed flowers or strobes composed of membranous scales. The scent is quirky and very friendly.

Taste: mildly astringent and highly bitter.

Medicinal parts: cones or strobes.

Solvents: Water to boil, alcohol to dilute.

Bodily influence: tonic, diuretic, tense, anodyne, anthelmintic, hypnotic, febri-fuge, sedative.

Uses: This ancient herb, in certain situations, is an excellent user. In cough syrups where there is nervousness, and in heart palpitation, ten drops' fluid extract is also used. Hop decoction cleanses the blood, making it effective for venereal in-fections and skin disorders of all sorts, such as swelling, ringworm, creeping sores, tetters, and discoloration. It can tone the liver, make the gallbladder become slow, and improve urinary production. Used primarily for a sedative or hypnotic ac-tion, sleep generation, restlessness reduction, and pain relief, particularly if com-bined with chamomile flowers.

Used internally as well as externally.

In delirium tremens, nervous fatigue, fear, worms, and lupulin tincture, it does not disorder the stomach or induces constipation. It is also effective in after-pains and in minimizing gonorrhoea discomfort.

Dose: one teaspoonful of flowers to 1 cupful of boiling water, sliced small or granulated. During the day, drink one cupful of ice, a big mouthful at a time. 5–20 minims of the tincture.

Note: An ointment formed by boiling two parts of stramonium (jimsonweed) and one part of hops in lard is an excellent remedy for skin irritation and skin itching.

2.25. HYDRANGEA - *Hydrangea Macrophylla*

Family: *Hydrangeaceae*

Common Names: Hortensia, Hortensia de Virginie, Hortensia en Arbre, Wild Hydrangea.

Features: Hydrangea is a genus of about 100 flowering plant species native to North and South America and Southern and Eastern Asia (from Japan to China, the Himalayas and Indonesia). From early spring to late fall, hydrangeas bear flowers. Medicine is produced using the root and the rhizome (underground stem).

Uses: Hydrangea is used for conditions of the urinary tract, such as bowel, urethra, and prostate infections; swollen prostate; and kidney stones. It is used for hay fever as well. Hydrangea chemicals can induce increased urine production, which may help with some problems with the urinary tract.

Dose: The sufficient dose of hydrangea depends on a variety of factors, including the age, fitness, and many other circumstances of the patient. There is no research evidence at this time to establish an acceptable number of doses for hydrangea. Bear in mind that not always are natural products inherently healthy and dosages may be essential. Be sure to follow the required product label guidelines and contact the pharmacist or doctor or other healthcare provider before using them.

Cautions: Hydrangea, when taken by mouth for only a few days, is Probably Healthy for most people. Nausea, vomiting, diarrhoea, dizziness, and chest tightness are among the side effects.

Using over 2 grams of dried hydrangea rhizome / root at a time is possibly unhealthy. The use of hydrangea for long stretches of time is most possibly dangerous. For this mix, be careful. Lithium Contact Rating: Mild.

Hydrangea may have an effect like a "diuretic" or water pill. Taking hydrangea may reduce how well lithium gets out of the body. This could raise the amount of lithium in the body and contribute to significant side effects. If you are taking lithium, consult with your healthcare professional prior to using this medication. It may be appropriate to adjust the lithium dosage.

2.26. JUNIPER - *Juniperus Communis*

Family: *Cupressaceae*

Common names: Juniper bush, juniper berries.

Features: An ornamental evergreen of the pine family of around forty varieties of trees and shrubs. A smaller species, typically less than 25 feet high, is the common juniper, and many of its various varieties are less than 10 feet. This shrub is widespread from Canada south to Canada on dusty, barren hills.

Medicinal part: Ripe, dried berries.

Solvents: Water to simmer, marijuana.

Bodily influence: Diuretic, carminative, stimulant.

Uses: It is used with digestion issues, including stomach upset, abdominal gas, bloating, heartburn, lack of appetite, and infections of gastrointestinal (GI) and intestinal worms. It is sometimes used for infections of the urinary tract (UTIs) and stones of the kidneys and bladder. Treating diabetes, snakebite, and cancer are other uses.

For wounds and for inflammation in muscles and joints, certain individuals add juniper straight to the skin. Juniper essential oil is inhaled for treating the discomfort of bronchitis and numbness.

Dose: Several teaspoons of berries are normally prepared by maceration (softening by soaking) to create an infusion, and then added to 1 pint of boiling water for 1/2 hour or more. The mixture should be cooled and separated into four parts, and taken in the morning, midday, afternoon, and evening—a treatment of 10-30 drops of tincture.

Cautions: Cannot be used for irritation of the kidneys.

2.27. MULLEIN - *Verbascum*

Family: *Scrophulariaceae*

Common Names: Aaron's Rod, American Mullein, Adam's Flannel, Beggar's Blanket, Blanket Herb, Candlewick, Candle flower.

Dose: A variety of variables, such as the user's age, fitness, and many other factors, depending on the required dose of mullein. There is not adequate clinical evidence at this time to establish an acceptable dosage level for mullein.

Vintage illustration #14_Mullein

2.28. MAGNOLIA - *Magnolia Grandiflora*

Family: *Magnoliaceae*

Common Names: Beaver Tree, Xin Ye Hua, Xin Yi Hua.

Features: Magnolia is a plant. People use the bark and flower buds to make Medicine.

Uses: For weight loss, stomach disorders, constipation, inflammation, anxiety, stress, depression, flu, headache, stroke, and asthma, magnolia is used.
For stuffy nose, runny nose, common cold, sinus discomfort, hay fever, headache,

and dark facial spots, Magnolia flower bud is used.

For toothaches, certain individuals add magnolia flower buds directly to the gums.

Magnolia flower bud extract is used as a skin whitener in rub-on skin care products and to reduce or mitigate skin inflammation caused by the other components.

Magnolia bark is an ingredient of traditional Chinese and Japanese (Kampo) medicine of Hange-koboku-to, which consists of 5 plant extracts, and in Saiboku-to, which consists of 10 plant extracts. To relieve discomfort and nervous stress and to enhance sleep, these extracts are used. Some scholars claim that what makes these drugs work is honokiol, a compound in magnolia bark.

Magnolia appears to have behaviour in animals that decreases fear. It could also increase the body 's development of steroids to combat asthma. Both the magnolia study was in labs.

Sleepiness and drowsiness may be caused by alcohol. Sleepiness and drowsiness may also be caused by Magnolia bark. It could induce too much sleepiness to take large quantities of magnolia bark along with alcohol.

Dose: The adequate dose of magnolia depends on a variety of considerations, such as age, fitness and some other circumstances of the patient. There is not adequate clinical evidence available at this time to establish a reasonable range of doses for magnolia. Bear in mind that not always are natural products inherently healthy and dosages may be essential. Be sure to follow the required product label guidelines and contact the pharmacist or doctor or other healthcare provider before using them.

2.29. NETTLE - *Urtica Dioica*

Family: *Urticaceae*

Common Names: Bichu, Common Nettle, Graine d'Ortie, Feuille d'Ortie, Urticae Radix.

Medicinal Part: Stinging nettle is a plant. The above-ground parts and roots are utilized as Medicine.

Uses: For osteoarthritis and diabetes, the Stinging Nettle is used. It is often used for infections of the urinary tract (UTIs), kidney stones, swollen prostate gland, muscle discomfort, among other disorders. However, to confirm these applications, there is no strong scientific research.

Diabetes. In persons with type II diabetes, having stinging nettle leaf prep for 8 to 12 weeks tends to decrease blood sugar.

Osteoarthritis. In individuals with osteoarthritis, having stinging nettle leaf prep by mouth or applying them to the skin can relieve discomfort. The need for pain killers could also be minimized by having stinging nettle leaf prep by mouth. Ingredients that could minimize inflammation and improve urinary output are found in Stinging nettle.

Interactions: With stinging nettle Lithium Interacts. Diabetes medicines (Antidiabetic drugs) interact with stinging nettle. High blood pressure medications (antihypertensive drugs) interact with stinging nettle. The interaction of sedative drugs (CNS depressants) with stinging nettle. The interaction of Warfarin (Coumadin) with stinging nettle

Dose: Scientific research has tested the following doses (for adults):

For diabetes: for 12 weeks, stinging nettle 500 mg leaf extract was taken three times every day by mouth. For 8 weeks, 3.3 g of stinging nettle leaf was also taken three times every day. Also used was a mixed formula comprising stinging nettle 200 mg, milk thistle 200 mg, and frankincense 200 mg given three times a day for three months.

For osteoarthritis: daily use of crude stinging nettle leaf 9 g. An infusion having stinging nettle leaf 5 mg and diclofenac 50 mg every day for 14 days was also taken. For 12 weeks, a particular combination product (medAgil Gesundheitsgesellschaft mbH, Rosaxan) comprising stinging nettle, devil's claw, rosehip, and Vit D was taken by mouth at 40 mL daily was used.

For osteoarthritis, fresh stinging nettle leaves were applied to damaged joints once a day for 30 seconds for one week. For 2 weeks, a particular cream comprising leaf extract of stinging nettle was also used twice every day.

Caution: <u>Pregnancy/breastfeeding, diabetes, and low blood pressure: people with renal issues must use it with caution.</u>

2.30. OREGON GRAPE - *Mahonia Aquifolium*

Family: *Berberidaceae*

Common Names: Holly-leaf barberry, Oregon grape holly, mountain grape, Oregon barberry, blue barberry, Mahonia.

Features: It is a therapeutic herb. Much before the Europeans and other settlers started moving in. The plant has also been used for appetite enhancement in indigenous societies. Today, it is widely used as a replacement for goldenseal, which has similar antimicrobial properties and is now known to be an endangered species owing to over-harvesting.

Medicinal part: The roots (golden yellow) of the plant are utilized for its medicinal properties

Uses: Indigenous tribes of America used the Oregon grape for several illnesses, including fever, jaundice, arthritis, diarrhoea, among other illnesses.

The Oregon grape root has been used to cure numerous illnesses, including colds, flu, hepatitis, herpes, syphilis, upset stomach, tumours, skin conditions, yeast infections, and much more, as herbal medication.

The usage of Oregon grape has been touted by herbalists, saying it successfully stimulates liver activity, cures illnesses, and improves digestive health.

In patients with insulin intolerance, it has been found to reduce blood sugar. It has cholesterol-lowering properties as well.

Oregon Grape is considered to have antifungal and antibacterial effects as an alkaloid derivative of several herbs, including barberry, goldenseal, and other plants. It is known that alkaloids help in battling different kinds of infections. It has been used to relieve problems such as diarrhoea, persistent candidiasis, and more.

In a skin disease called psoriasis, Oregon grape is often known to reduce the immature skin cells overproduction and decrease inflammation.

Interactions: Some drugs can interact with the Oregon grape but might conflict with the body's ability to break down certain forms of liver medications.

Examples of drugs with which Oregon grape should not be taken include:

• Cyclosporine (Neoral, Sandimmune)

- Doxycycline
- Tetracycline
- Any medications that are changed by the liver

Dose: It has been used as a tea widely by boiling few teaspoons (5 to 15 g) of chopped roots in two cups (500 millilitres) of water for 15 mins, then cooling & straining the mixture

Though further tests are required to ensure Oregon grape ingestion protection, herbalists suggest that no more than three cups (750 ml) of tea should be drunk every day.

It is used as a tincture, an alcohol-based herbal blend, supplied at 1/2 - 3/4 teaspoon (3 millilitres) doses and taken per day three times.

A particular mixture of 10 percent extract cream of Oregon grape bark is commercially manufactured as a topical psoriasis cream by a company called Relieva, to be applied to the infected region (around 2 months) of the skin two-three times per day. Often available are creams with a 10 percent Oregon grape root tincture.

Caution: Some drugs can interact with the Oregon grape but might conflict with the body's ability to break down certain forms of liver medications.

Examples of drugs with which Oregon grape should not be taken include: Cyclosporine (Neoral, Sandimmune)' Doxycycline, Tetracycline. Any medications that are changed by the liver.

2.31. PRIMROSE (EVENING) - Oenothera Biennis

Family: *Onagraceae*

Common Names: Aceite de Onagra, Cis-Linoleic Acid, Acide Cis-linoléique,EPO, Evening Primrose, Primrose Oil, Scabish, Sun Drop.

Features: A plant common to South and North America is the evening primrose. It is also rising all over Europe and Asia (parts). It has yellow colour flowers that open at sunset and shut during the day.

Medicinal Part: The seeds oil of evening primrose are utilized.

Uses: For premenstrual syndrome (PMS), menopausal symptoms, swelling, arthritis, and other disorders, evening primrose is used, but no good clinical data is there to justify its use.

Evening primrose oil is also used in foods as an essential fatty acids source.

In the production sector, evening primrose oil is being used in cosmetics and soaps. Evening primrose used to be licensed in Britain to relieve eczema and breast discomfort. The MCA (Medicines Control Agency), the British counterpart to the FDA, has revoked licenses for evening primrose drugs sold for these applications as prescription drugs.

Damage to nerves induced by diabetes. The study suggests that the regular consumption of evening primrose oil for 6 to 12 months enhances the effects of diabetes-induced nerve injury. Osteoporosis. In elderly people with osteoporosis, having evening primrose oil with calcium and fish oil reduces bone loss and improves bone density. There are "fatty acids" in evening primrose oil. Certain women experiencing breast pain do not have large enough amounts of these "fatty acids." Fatty acids often tend to help alleviate inflammation associated with disorders like arthritis and eczema.

Interactions: Antiplatelet/Anticoagulant drugs Medications that delay blood clotting interfere with evening primrose oil.

Anaesthesia medications used during the surgery interacts with the evening primrose oil.phenothiazines interact with the evening primrose oil.

Dose: For Breast pain: 3 to 4 g daily.

2.32. PURSLANE - *Portulaca Oleracea*

Family: *Portulacaceae*

Common Names: Ma Chi Xian, Garden (common) purslane, Munyeroo, Portulaca, Pourpier, Purslane, Pigweed, Rigla, Sormai

Uses: It is used as fatty acid (omega 3) vegetable source and is rich in minerals and vitamins. It has a pronounced antioxidant function. Roles are indicated in type II diabetes, oral lichen planus asthma, and uterine bleeding, but few and complex clinical trials are, in fact.

Dose: For dosage recommendations, few clinical trials are available; however, 180-milligram purslane extract per day has been tested in diabetic patients, & powdered seeds were taken at 1-30 grams daily in doses divided, also ethanol & aqueous purslane extracts. For a number of indications, traditional Chinese medicine guidelines have been recorded for 9 - 15 grams of dried aerial pieces and 10 - 30 g of fresh herbs. Around 300 - 400 mg, alpha-linolenic acid produces one hundred g of purslane leaves.

2.33. PASSIONFLOWER - *Passiflora Incarnata*

Family: *Passifloraceae*

Common Names: Apricot Vine, Wild Passionflower, Water Lemon.

Uses: Some evidence suggests that taking flowers of passion by mouth will decrease anxiety symptoms. It could potentially function as well as other prescription drugs.

Anxiousness before surgery. Some studies show that when taken 30-90 minutes prior to surgery, taking passionflower by mouth can decrease anxiety before surgery. It may potentially function as well as any other pre-operative anxiety medications, such as melatonin or midazolam.

Interactions: Sedative drugs (CNS depressants) are associated with passionflower.

Sleepiness and drowsiness can be caused by the passionflower. Sedatives are called drugs that induce sleepiness. It might induce too much sleepiness to take passionflower along with sedative drugs.

Pentobarbital (Nembutal), phenobarbital (Luminal), secobarbital (Seconal), clonazepam (Klonopin), lorazepam (Ativan), zolpidem (Ambien) and others are used in some sedative medicines.

Dose: Clinical research has tested the following doses.

For Adults by mouth. For 2-8 weeks, capsules containing 400 mg of passion flower extract were used twice daily for anxiety. In addition, 45 drops of passion flower liquid extract were used every day for up to one month.

20 drops of a particular passionflower extract taken the night before surgery and 90 minutes before the beginning of surgery were used to alleviate anxiety before surgery. Tablets of this medication were also taken at a dosage of 500 mg 90 minutes before the start of the procedure. Passionflower 260 mg taken 30 minutes prior to dental surgery, or 1000 mg of passionflower taken one hour prior to surgery. Also, 30 minutes prior to surgery, 5 mL of syrup containing 700 mg of passionflower extract (Passiflora syrup by Sandoz) was taken.

2.34. RED CLOVER - *Trifolium Pratense*

Family: *Legumes*

Common Names: Beebread, Clovone, Cow Clover, Daidzein, Genistein, Isoflavone, Meadow Clover

Features: The red clover is a seedling. The blossoms are used to manufacture medicine. Red clover is prescribed for menopausal complications, frail and delicate muscles, elevated cholesterol levels, and many other disorders, but no good clinical data is sufficient to support these applications. Red clover is used as a flavouring component in meats and drinks. Red clover contains molecules which are similar to the hormone estrogen, or phytoestrogens.

Uses: Enlarged (benign prostatic hyperplasia or BPH) prostate. Any early literature shows that some effects of an enlarged prostate may be relieved by red clover supplements. It tends to minimise urination at night.

There is some early evidence that red clover could help alleviate the discomfort and tenderness of cyclic breast pain.

Menopausal signs. Most tests indicate that taking red clover by mouth would not alleviate symptoms such as hot flashes for up to a year. But some evidence suggests that taking a particular red clover substance (Promensil, Novogen) could decrease the occurrence of hot flashes. Some studies show that the use of red clover can improve vaginal dryness. Other study has also found that red clover can enhance menopausal psychiatric symptoms, such as depression and anxiety. Yet not all review approves.

Possibly ineffective for poor and brittle (osteoporosis) bones. The majority of evidence indicates that the frequent use of red clover does not increase bone density in women.

Insufficient evidence for baldness in male-pattern (androgenic alopecia). Early research suggests that in individuals with hair loss, applying a combination product containing red clover flower extract may improve hair growth.

Large serum levels (hyperlipidaemia) of cholesterol or other fats (lipids). Most evidence suggests that in women who have significantly elevated cholesterol lev

Vintage illustration #19_Red Clover

els, taking red clover extracts by mouth for 3 months to a year does not decrease low-density lipoprotein (LDL or "bad") cholesterol or raise high-density lipoprotein (HDL or "good") cholesterol levels.

More evidence is needed to rate red clover for these uses: Asthma, eczema (atopic dermatitis), breast cancer,

swelling (inflammation) of the main airways in the lung (bronchitis), burns, cough, indigestion (dyspepsia), cancer of the lining of the uterus (endometrial cancer), premenstrual syndrome (PMS), sexually transmitted diseases (STDs), scaly, itchy skin (psoriasis), whooping cough (pertussis), wound healing.

When applied in therapeutic quantities to the skin, red clover is probably healthy.

Dose: The required dosage of red clover depends on a variety of variables, such as age, weight, and some other factors of the user. There is not adequate clinical evidence at this time to establish the optimal range of doses for red clover. Bear in mind that not always are natural products inherently healthy and dosages may be essential. Be sure to follow the required product label guidelines and contact the pharmacist or doctor or other healthcare provider before using them.

Interactions: Moderate interaction.

Medications changed by the liver (Cytochrome P450 2C19 (CYP2C19) substrates) interacts with Red Clover. Some medications are changed and broken down by the liver. Red clover might decrease how quickly the liver breaks down some medications. Taking red clover along with some medications that are broken down by the liver can increase the effects and side effects of some medications. Before taking red clover, talk to your healthcare provider if you take any medications that are changed by the liver. Some medications that are changed by the liver include omeprazole (Prilosec), lansoprazole (Prevacid), and pantoprazole (Protonix); diazepam (Valium); carisoprodol (Soma); nelfinavir (Viracept); and others.

Birth control pills (Contraceptive drugs) interacts with red Clover. Some birth control pills contain estrogen. Red clover might have some of the same effects as estrogen. But red clover isn't as strong as the estrogen in birth control pills. Taking red clover along with birth control pills might decrease the effectiveness of birth control pills. If you take birth control pills along with red clover, use an additional form of birth control such as a condom.

Some birth control pills include ethinyl estradiol and levonorgestrel (Triphas-il), ethinyl estradiol and norethindrone (Ortho-Novum 1/35, Ortho-Novum 7/7/7), and others.

Estrogens interacts with Red Clover. Large amounts of red clover might have some of the same effects as estrogen. But red clover isn't as strong as estrogen pills. Taking red clover along with estrogen pills might decrease the effects of estrogen pills. Some estrogen pills include conjugated equine estrogens (Premarin), ethinyl estradiol, estradiol, and others.

Medications changed by the liver (Cytochrome P450 1A2 (CYP1A2) substrates) interacts with Red Clover. Some medications are changed and broken down by the liver. Red clover might decrease how quickly the liver breaks down some medications. Taking red clover along with some medications that are broken down by the liver can increase the effects and side effects of some medications. Before taking red clover, talk to your healthcare provider if you take any medications that are changed by the liver. Some medications that are changed by the liver include amitriptyline (Elavil), haloperidol (Haldol), ondansetron (Zofran), propranolol (Inderal), theophylline (Theo-Dur, others), verapamil (Calan, Isoptin, others), and others.

Caution: For most people, red clover is likely harmless when consumed by mouth in the proportions found in food. It is probably healthy in therapeutic quantities when used. In certain women, red clover can cause rashes, muscle pain, fever, nausea, and vaginal bleeding (spotting).

Be cautious with this combination.

Pregnancy and breast-feeding. When eaten by mouth in concentrations typically found in food, red clover is possibly healthy. When used in therapeutic quantities, though, it is possibly dangerous. During pregnancy or breast-feeding, red clover behaves like oestrogen and could disrupt major hormone balances. Using it not.

Bleeding disorders. The risk of bleeding may be raised by red clover. Stop massive numbers and use them with caution.

Hormone-sensitive disorders such as cancer of the breast, cancer of the prostate, cancer of the ovary, endometriosis, or fibroids of the prostate: Red clover may function like estrogen. Don't use red clover if you have some disorder that could be made worse by estrogen.

Protein S deficiency. Individuals with a deficiency in protein S have an elevated chance in blood clots developing. There is some doubt that in these individuals, red clover may increase the risk of clot formation because it has some of the effects of estrogen. If you have protein S deficiency, don't use the red clover.

Surgery: Red clover could delay coagulation of blood. During and after surgery, it may increase the risk of bleeding. Avoid taking the red clover at least 2 weeks before the surgery is scheduled.

2.38. VALERIAN - *Valeriana Officinalis*

Family: *Valerianaceae*

Common Names: Amantilla, All-Heal, Belgium Valerian, Baldrian, Baldrian-wurzel, Common Valerian

Features: It is originally from Europe and Asia (some parts) but is now rising in North America.

For sleep disorders, particularly insomnia (inability to sleep), Valerian is more widely used. Valerian is often used orally for psychological stress and anxiety.

In processing, valerian extracts and oil are used as flavourings in foods and drinks.

Medicinal Part: Root.

Uses: Insomnia. Although there is some contradictory evidence, most studies suggest that taking Valerian will decrease by around 15 to 20 mins the period it takes to fall asleep. Often, Valerian appears to boost the quality of sleep. Valerian extract doses of 400 to 900 mg taken up to 2 hrs prior to sleep appear to perform best. Before an impact is apparent, consistent usage for many days, perhaps up to one month, can be required. Some reports indicate that Valerian can help enhance sleep when mixed with other herbs, like lemon and balm hops. Valerian can also boost the standard of sleep of persons who refrain from the usage of sleeping tablets. However, some evidence shows that Valerian doesn't really cure insomnia as easily as "sleeping tablets."

Menopausal symptoms. Research suggests that in postmenopausal women, taking 675 to 1060 mg of valerian root every day for eight weeks will reduce the frequency and intensity of hot flashes.

Valerian appears to be working on the brain & nervous system as a sedative.

When administered by mouth regularly for 4 to 8 weeks, Valerian is safe for kids.

Interactions: Liver-changed drugs (substrates of Cytochrome P450 3A4 (CYP3A4)) interact with Valerian.

Such liver-changed drugs include lovastatin (Mevacor), itraconazole (Sporanox), ketoconazole (Nizoral), triazolam (Halcion), fexofenadine (Allegra), and many more.

Dose: Insomnia. 400-900 mg of valerian extract for around six weeks before bedtime, or 120 mg of valerian extract, lemon balm extract 80 mg for up to 30 days or up to 30 days before bedtime.

374 of 500 mg valerian extract + 83.8 to 120 mg hop extract for 2 to 4 weeks before bedtime, or 300 mg valerian extract, passionflower extract 80 mg, and 30 mg of hop extract for up to two weeks before bedtime. Take Valerian 30 mins to 2 hours until bedtime.

For menopause symptoms. For eight weeks, 225 mg ground valerian root was taken three times every day. Even for eight weeks, 530 mg valerian root extract was taken twice every day.

Caution: Inadequate knowledge is available about the protection of Valerian during pregnancy/breastfeeding. For most adults, Valerian is SAFE when consumed by mouth and used in short-term medicinal doses. It is not clear regarding the efficacy of long-term usage.

2.39. WORMWOOD - *Artemisia Absinthium*

Family: *Asteraceae*

Common names: Absinthe, Absinth, Absinthii Herba, Absinthe Suisse, Absinthites, Absinthium.

Medicinal Part: The plant above-ground parts and oil are used.

Uses: It is used for numerous disorders of digestion, such as lack of appetite, gastrointestinal upset, intestinal spasms, and disease of the gall bladder. It is also used to treat the liver's illness, depression, body pain, memory loss, worm infections, and fever, improve sexual desire, induce sweating, and as a tonic. For Crohn's disease and a kidney dysfunction termed IgA nephropathy, wormwood is used. Wormwood oil is often used to enhance the imagination, improve sexual desire, and for digestive disorders.

For osteoarthritis (OA), and for curing wounds and bug bites, certain people apply it directly to the body. To relieve pain, its oil is used as a counterirritant.

When consumed by mouth, wormwood is Harmless in the concentrations typically used in food and drinks, including vermouth and bitters, as long as these items are thujone-free.

Dose: The required dosage of wormwood depends on a number of variables, such as age, fitness, and some other factors of the user. There is not adequate clinical evidence at this point to establish the optimal doses range for wormwood.

Interactions: Medications used to stop Anticonvulsants (seizures) interact with Wormwood

Caution: When ingested by mouth during pregnancy, wormwood is Possibly Unhealthy in concentrations greater than typically present in food. Kidney problems: Taking wormwood oil can induce failure of the kidneys.

Epilepsy and seizure disorders: Wormwood includes thujone, which may induce seizures. There is fear that in people who are vulnerable to them, wormwood may make seizures more probable.

2.40. WITCH HAZEL - *Hamamelis Virginiana*

Family: *Hamamelidaceae*

Common Names: Café du Diable, Avellano de Bruja, Hamamelis, Hamamélis de Virginie, Hamamélis, Hamamelis virginiana, Hazel,

Features: It is a deciduous tree or shrub native to North America, and is now planted in Europe and Asia as well. The shrub can reach a height of 4.6 m (15 ft). In the autumn, it flowers, producing bright yellow flowers. Medicine is used to make the leaves, bark, and twigs. You will see a substance (Hamamelis water, purified witch hazel extract) called witch hazel water. It is a solvent distilled from witch hazel's dried stems, bark, and partly dormant twigs.

Witch hazel leaf extract, bark extract, and witch hazel water are used as astringents in processing to tighten the flesh. In certain drugs, they are often used to give certain items the potential to slow down or avoid bleeding. Insect bites, stings, teething, haemorrhoids, swelling, irritations, and mild discomfort are handled with these drugs.

Uses: The application of witch hazel water to the skin can help to temporarily alleviate haemorrhoids and other anal disorders from scratching, inflammation, pain, and burning.

Mild bleeds. The application to the skin of witch hazel bark, herb, or water eliminates moderate bleeding.

Inflammation of the skin. It appears that adding witch hazel cream relieves moderate skin inflammation, but not hydrocortisone as well. Other evidence suggests that the application to the skin of a particular witch hazel ointment (Hametum) tends to relieve signs of skin damage or sore skin as effectively as a childhood dexpanthenol ointment.

Witch hazel contains tannins called chemicals. Witch hazel can help minimise bleeding, help heal damaged skin, and kill bacteria when added directly to the skin.

Kids: Witch hazel, when added directly to the eyes, is likely healthy for kids.

Dose: Clinical research has tested the following doses.

For skin irritation in adults: A 10 percent witch hazel water after-sun lotion was used.

For skin irritation in children aged 2-11 years. An ointment containing witch hazel was applied multiple times a day.

Applied to the rectum. Witch hazel water was administered up to 6 times a day or after a bowel movement for scratching and pain associated with haemorrhoids and other anal disorders. Suppositories were implanted 1-3 times a day into the anus.

Caution: Witch hazel, when actually added to the skin, is LIKELY healthy for most adults. It might cause mild skin irritation in some individuals.

CONCLUSION

The Native American belief in the interconnectedness of human beings and nature is difficult to explain. As ancestors, all part of one large and at least theoretically prosperous family, they looked at all living things, as well as some physical facets of nature, such as rivers, mountains, and climates. We share our breath with everyone that is obvious, writes Native American psychotherapist Robert Blackwolf Jones, the deer, fox, hawk, lizard, tree and shark. The Native American philosopher Chief Seattle shares a similar sentiment, writing: "Man did not weave the web of life, he is merely a thread in it, so that whatever he does to the web, he does to himself."

The Native Americans claimed that a poor interaction with some facets of nature also induced illness. While there were clear explanations for certain forms of injury, such as snake bites and burns, it was difficult to describe internal diseases. The Native Americans thought that the angry spirits of animals, who took vengeance for insults they got in childhood, were more likely to cause "invisible" diseases. "An animal ghost will cause problems if reverence is not given to the body after it has been murdered," according to historian William Corlett. Since Native Americans assumed that humans and nature were closely connected, nearly any thought or behaviour might have negative effects if it displayed contempt for nature. For instance, spitting on a fire could rage the spirits and result in disease.

Nature, of course, has not always been regarded with apprehension. Much as when they were angry, the spirits of animals and other facets of nature could be dangerous, they might also be beneficial when they were happy. For one, the Native Americans believed that herbs and even animals' organs were full of enormous healing powers. During their various curing rituals, they also called on the spirits of animals for help. It was believed that various species had special characteristics and qualities, such as cunning, intellect, and courage. During healing rituals, Native Americans may call for individual animal spirits, asking each in return to share their special gifts with the person being healed. Still, of course, doctors are unlikely to consider calling on the spirits of eagles and bears to regulate blood pressure or cure arthritis, but depending on how it is handled, they are very mindful of nature's ability to cure or hurt. For example, prolonged exposure to sunlight can cause cancer, but when the sun is used properly (approximately 15 minutes of everyday exposure), it makes the body produce vitamin D, which is necessary for healthy bones. Nutrients are filled with the foods we consume, such as vitamin A, iron, folate, and sodium are important to life in right quantity; in abundance, all of them can be dangerous. Since the keys to wellbeing are peace and order, who does not benefit from learning a lesson from the Native American people? The way to start is by treating with the highest regard the world around us. "It's time we climbed down from the lonely pedestal we've made for ourselves, according to Robert Blackwolf Jones, and we remember our position alongside our fellow inhabitants."

NATIVE AMERICAN
HERBAL
DISPENSATORY

The medicine-making guide
for common ailments & radiant health

INTRODUCTION

Healing traditions of Native Americans enjoy a very long and rich history that extends far beyond recorded history. In the U.S. colonization, there is an increased attentiveness to medicinal botanicals as part of alternative medicines. In particular, Native American communities are becoming conscious of using herbals by both practitioners and consumers; many botanicals marketed nowadays as dietary supplements in the western world were used for similar motives by Native Americans. However, these supplements make up a number of the > 2500 different vascular taxa plant species and > 2800 species of all taxa known to have been coveted by the native populations of the continent North America for their medicinal properties. Cultures around the globe have relied on traditional natural medicine since ancient times to fulfill their health requirements. The global market for herbal remedies is on the rise, amid the modern age's technological and medical advances. This industry is expected to gross about $60 billion yearly.

Native American healing activities illustrate essential cultural perspectives and impact the formation of Native American people's culture. Such healing practices are based on perspectives and traditions that are generally outside the norm of Western psychological values but can profoundly affect the Native American sense of well-being. According to Hammerschlag, the ritual celebration of Native

Americans aims to invest symbolic significance in one's life experiences.

For their medicinal plant knowledge, Native Americans are acclaimed. Since seeing animals consuming such plants when they were ill, it is believed that they first began using plants and herbs for healing. The medicine men used to select every third plant they find to protect these plants against over-harvesting. Native Americans had a spiritual outlook on life. A person should have a sense of meaning and follow a fair, harmonious, and balanced course in life to be healthy. They thought that certain diseases were life lessons that the individual needed to learn and not intervene. The Native American interpretation of the various plants and herbs they have used for thousands of years is based on many modern medicines and remedies.

Native American Tradition

CHAPTER 1

with the usage of animal and plant substances and other practical procedures. Many healers have often used cups or suction tubes and purification and purging in addition to herbal remedies.

People in medicine have also been born into a family of several generations of people in medicine. Some might have the vision that inspired them to study this. In any scenario, until they became qualified to act alone, anyone who desired to be healers must first spend a long traineeship with some experienced medicine individual. The healers used the tools made from nature, such as skins, fur shells, bone, crystals, feathers, and root. Feathers were also used to take the Great Spirit's message, connected to the air and wind. In some cases, the healer can enter a state of trance and obtain the aid of "spirit guides."

In a bundle of medicine, made of hiding or cloth, which was securely tied, healers held their remedies and tools. Different bundles types were used for special purposes, like ceremonies and festivals: the healer's bundles, the tribe's, and bundles. The bundle of medicine contents is sacred, and it is normally forbidden to inquire regarding the personal bundle content. Due to the power they carried to nourish & nurture the group, medicine bundles leading to tribes were often named 'grandmothers.' Medicine pipes, which reflect the ebb & flow of life, are sometimes used in medicine bundles. The smoke exhaled is believed to carry prayers to the spirit. An aspect of individual healing methods is that it's regarded as a personal matter among the patient and the healer. Furthermore, the patient's interests are still valued within his/her cultural values.

1.3 HEALING RITUALS AND CEREMONIES

To bring the participants into peace with themselves, their environment, and tribe, symbolic healing rituals and ceremonies are also conducted. Ceremonies are utilized, but not used for human healing, to assist groups of individuals back to harmony. Some tribes, like the Navajo and Sioux, utilized a medicine wheel, sing, dance, and sacred hoop in rituals that could last for some days, varying widely from tribe to tribe.

Healers could also use painting, dancing, drumming, changing, feathers, and rattles for persons in the rituals of them. Stones (sacred) were often rubbed on the different parts of the human body.

Native Americans also used sweat baths or sweat lodges for purification and purging. It was often thought to remove evils and revitalize the body, used for balancing and healing. These baths range from just lying in the scorching sun under a blanket to little conical structures covered by branches and hides/blankets. With water, hot stones were covered within the lodge to make the steam bath, and the healer could pray, drum, or sing together for purifying the spirit here.

Sweat lodges have been used for various purposes, often merely to heal a person, sometimes before spiritual ceremonies for larger numbers of people or bringing clarity to an issue. The sage, the best cleansing herb, burnt in certain civilizations till it smoldered and let out smoke clouds. On the skin, It was smudged and was supposed to purify the soul and body, called "sweeping the smoke."

1.4 RELIGIOUS RIGHTS BANNING

The Federal Govt. started to ban the religious rights of Native Americans at the beginning of 1882, which influenced their medical methods. Due to their "great hindrance to civilization," the Interior Secretary of U.S, Henry Teller, requested to end all "Ceremonies and heathenish dances" on reservations. Hiram Price further supported this, Indian Affairs Commissioner, when 1883 report of his stated that there's no reasonable excuse why should an Indian be able to engage in practices that are repugnant to morality and decency, and ensuring better order on reservations requires that such active steps must be taken to avoid and, if necessary, put an end to the effect of demoralizing heathenish rites.

Efforts like these to eliminate Native American traditions result in the Wounded Knee Massacre on 29 December 1890, when attempted to ban by government "Ghost Dance" practice, a movement far-reaching that nonviolent prophesied end to the white American preached and expansion. Goals of Native Americans of living clean, cross-cultural assistance, and honest life. About 150 Native American men, women, and children were killed when the 7th Cavalry of U.S. was sent to the Lakota Sioux Rosebud and Pine Ridge Reserves to interrupt the participants' dance to be arrested. While charges were raised against the 7th Calvary participants for killing innocent people, all were found innocent. Two years later, when Thomas J. Morgan, Indian Affairs Commissioner ordered to sentences of around six months in jail for anyone who repeatedly engaged in religious dances/ served as men of medicine, more actions were taken to suppress religious practices. Native Americans focused on their medication for both injuries and illnesses before 1900. At the start 20th century, that began to shift when the IHS (Indian Health Service) opened hospitals and clinics. Although the spiritual harmony old traditions remained part of the community, many of the Native Americans start to utilize modern medicine, particularly in healing diseases of "white-man" for which no medicine was available to their healers.

After 1978, the Religious Freedom Act of American Indian passage, the ban against Native American spiritual practices remained in place. Unfortunately, much of the healing practices of Native Americans were completely forgotten or driven underground because of the ban.

Today, several tribes prefer to protect their people's knowledge of medicine, and this will not explore the idea with the non-Indians. A few claims that the exchange of healing knowledge would weaken medicine's spiritual power.

1.5 AMERICAN MEDICINE TODAY

Today's medical theory wave has started to shift back to a viewpoint that considers and respects each individual part, including their spiritual and mental states. Due to this, with natives and non-natives alike, the medical practices of Native Americans have again become popular. Many are cautious about pharmaceutical products' addictive properties, toxicity, and side effects and are moving to natural herbal cures. Quality Native American products also have been produced and used to cope with different illnesses for several decades. Although not necessarily accurate, herbal remedies like to be much less toxic than certain prescription drugs and have many less unpleasant side effects. Look for carefully formulated and controlled products that use strict pharmaceutical production levels and the best quality organic ingredients while choosing herbal remedies. Herbal products can be handled properly, much like every other medication. In the appropriate version, at the appropriate dosage level, obey the directions, and use them.

CHAPTER 2

Vintage illustration #1_Cabbage

1. ABSCESS AND GINGIVITIS

Abscesses and boils which develop under the skin are swollen, red, pus-filled bumps. They are sometimes painful because they keep on growing until they are removed. Bacteria that invade, and then incite hair follicles causes boils. They can expand to the length of a baseball, and they can be red and sore in the region around the skin, too.

You're not supposed to pick at or pinch a boil. It could invade surrounding areas or drive the infection further into the skin and further boil if it is not appropriately drained.

Indian Sorrel Leaves (Sarvajjaya)
Make Indian Sorrel Leave Poultice (Sarvajjaya). Apply twice a day on the impacted portion day.
OR: Pound out some new leaves. Add a tiny volume of hot water. Multiple times a day, apply the paste.

Aloe Vera (Gheekumari)
Apply the crushed leaves to the infected region
OR: On the injured portion, put the pulp and bandage.

Cabbage
Take up the Cabbage Leaf. After eliminating the ridges, dip it in hot water. Apply it like a poultice. Put a flexible bandage in the spot. Frequently Replace the leaf.

Echinacea
For 5-10 days, drink two times a day.
OR: The root decoction is packed. Drink three times a day.

Fenugreek (Methi)
By boiling six teaspoons of Fenugreek seed in water (1 cup), prepare a poultice for 5 to 7 minutes.
Three drops of the thyme oil are added. Add a warm cloth to the infected region and protect it. Repeat the process 3-4 times a day.

Tea Tree Essential Oil For Abscess

Add 2 to 3 Tea Tree oil drops to a teaspoon of water. The impacted section is washed 4 to 5 times a day. It will kill the bacteria.

Or: Add Tea Tree oil a few drops to a cotton swab, then apply it to the infected area a few times a day.

More Recipes

1. Prepare the Mullein poultice (three parts) & Lobelia poultice (one part). Apply it to the region concerned.

2. Prepare one onion poultice with five cloves of garlic. Apply it to the Abscess

3. Take basil leaves half a cup and crushed Vetiver roots half a cup. Dip them up overnight in a boiled water jug. Have it all day.

4. Take an equal amount of scraps from Vetiver and Sandalwood. Together, grind them. In Rosewater, mix one tsp of powder and add it once a day. OR: Smash any scraps from Vetiver and Sandalwood. Dip for 2 hrs in a water-containing mud pot. Frequently Drink it.

5. Combine Sandalwood, Vetiver and Turmeric powder in similar amounts. Add a little water, then apply it to the impacted section.

6. Take the flowers of Woodfordia Fruticosa (Dhawai). Camel Thorn (Javasa) oil blend. Hold it there, for 10 -15 min on a medium flame. Apply the impacted section lukewarmly.

7. Take a teaspoon of Bush Grape (Amalbel) root powder and 1/4 of a teaspoon of Black pepper. By adding a tiny volume of water, Create a paste. Apply twice a day on the impacted portion for 20 mins a day.

8. Add one teaspoon of lime juice to a bottle of Sour Gourd juice. When empty stomach, drink it. This improves boils filled with blood.

Poultices For Inflammation

The following are herbs with healing properties that can be used for a number of illnesses, such as mild skin irritations/abrasions, to produce poultices:

- Turmeric
- Ginger
- Garlic
- Onion
- Dandelion
- Eucalyptus
- Cat's Claw

How Poultice Is Made

For problems such as slight skin irritations or wounds, bruises, or moderate discomfort from arthritis or some minor injury, you can obtain relief from the homemade poultice.

Poultice of herbs

To produce a poultice of herbs that can be used to treat mild pain, abrasions, and more.

WHAT YOU'RE GOING TO NEED
1 tsp turmeric powder 1 ounce of ginger, finely chopped/grated 1/4 thin-sliced raw onion 1 garlic clove chopped 2 tsp coconut oil Cheesecloth/bandage of cotton

Vintage illustration #2_Black Pepper Branch

Instructions

1. In a pan on low heat, the coconut oil is added, followed by the remaining ingredients, and permit it to heat till it is almost dried but not burnt.

2. Turn the stove off and move the ingredients to some bowl for cooling to make it warm.

3. Lay flat the cloth, and the mixture is added to the middle of the fabric

4. To create the pack or collect it, fold the fabric twice and attach it with a string/rubber band to make a handle; however, you want it until the ingredients remain within the fabric.

5. Place it for 20 mins on the affected area.

Castor Oil

Castor oil produces a molecule that is a normal yet potent anti-inflammatory, named ricinoleic acid. This makes it a perfect natural remedy for boils, in combination with its potent antibacterial effects. At least three times a day, add a tiny amount of castor oil directly to the area infected until it is healed completely.

Neem Oil

Neem oil, also referred to as Indian lilac, has antibacterial, antimicrobial, and antiseptic properties that rapidly cure skin infections. Apply the oil directly to a boil 3-4 times a day to cure boils. Before and after you apply the oil, ensure that you wash your hands.

Tea Tree Oil

The tea tree oil has good antiseptic and antibacterial effects, helping cure boil caused by a bacterial infection. As it may have a burning effect, Tea tree oil should not be added explicitly to the skin. With a tsp of coconut or olive oil, combine five drops of tea tree oil. Put it on a cotton swab and add it to the region 2-3 times per day. Do this regularly till the boil is fully out.

Turmeric Powder

Turmeric powder has anti-inflammatory and antibacterial effects, which will help cure a boil and quickly eliminate it. As a result, eastern medicine has been used as a natural blood purifier for thousands of years.You can opt to consume turmeric powder or use it to cure boils topically, or both. Boil a tsp of turmeric powder in milk or water and drink it until it is cooled, three times a day. Mix Turmeric with ginger or water to create a paste and apply it to the boil two times a day, to use it topically.

Gingivitis Treatments

Some natural treatments can help you deal with tooth pain and avoid worsening tooth infections. It would be best to use specific herbal therapies to manage the discomfort and prevent it from spreading and getting worse. Not all of these treatments would function for every human, but they will get you some comfort if you're in misery from an infected tooth.

Aloe Vera

Since it has powerful antibacterial qualities, Aloe Vera gel is mostly used to heal wounds and injuries, or skin irritations. Still, it is often an excellent way to relieve the discomfort of an infected tooth. It will help to treat abscesses in the gums as well. When you purchase Aloe Vera gel to be used on your mouth, consider buying Aloe Vera grade food to eat healthily. Aloe Vera liquid may still be used, although the cream can be added on the teeth and gums more quickly. For additional pain reliever, place the aloe vera bottle in the refrigerator. Immediate relief from pain and the added bonus of battling bacteria may be given by adding cold Aloe Vera gel to a sore swollen tooth or gum.

Coconut Oil Pulling

A very controversial method is oil pulling. Few individuals claim it helps to preserve proper oral health and advocate doing it regularly. There is no proof that pulling oil has any therapeutic advantages for oral health. Coconut oil has specific strong antibacterial effects, so it is likely that oil can either shorten the infection's length or make the effects more manageable by utilizing liquid coconut oil.

Essential oils

Essential oils are being used for decades for their healing effects. Essential oils are prepared from plants distilled with steam or water, or cold-pressed to obtain the plant's oil in stems and leaves. By far, steam distillation is the most popular modern way to extract oil from plants, but cold pressing was also used in earlier centuries to guarantee that the highest quality oil was produced.

Essential oils must be placed in a cool place, away from food or spices, to promote healing and alleviate pain. On a cotton swab or cotton ball, put a few drops of the oil and then apply it to your teeth.

USEFUL OILS IN TREATING A VARIETY OF DENTAL PROBLEMS, INCLUDING INFECTIONS

Thyme Oil
Clove Oil
Tea Tree Oil
Lavender Oil
Oregano Oil

Make sure you are using pure therapeutic grade essential oils. At every health food shop, you will find these. Certain grocery co-ops even offer them, and you can order them online. Shop from reputable labels who have a good quality rating. Double-check to ensure that the product states that the oil is medicinal and therapeutic grade. Most manufacturers use "natural" oils these days to make soups and perfumes. Those oils are scented oils but are not pure essential oils. Such oils have a little medicinal benefit and, if swallowed, may be toxic.

Garlic

A home cure for tooth abscesses that is easy to locate and cheap to purchase is garlic. The thought of smelling like garlic does not appeal to you only because you are attempting to cure a tooth, but garlic's curing benefits make it worth the scent. A compound named Allicin in fresh raw garlic can provide substantial pain reduction and antibacterial effects that can lessen or remove the infection in a tooth. If you think you have an infected tooth and cannot instantly go to the doctor, it can help. Slice a clove of garlic and softly bite it down with your infected tooth. You may need to leave a slice of garlic against your teeth for a few minutes to make it successful.

Herbal Teas

Herbal tea, for several common illnesses, is another time-tested home cure. By obtaining the leaves and stems of different herbs and merely soaking them in hot water to produce a tea, you may make your herbal teas. However, buying medicinal grade teas that are already manufactured would likely be more successful.

A better herb content and a better dosage would contain good quality therapeutic grade teas to be more effective. If your teeth are heat sensitive due to the infection, brew the tea, and let it steep for up to fifteen minutes depending on how you like it to be, and then let it cool to average room temperature until you drink it.

To help ease the effects of a tooth infection, Fenugreek is a common tea. Simultaneously, not enough study has been conducted to show that its medicinal properties are useful for home treatment of tooth infection. In most health food stores and certain grocery stores with an alternative health food portion or alternative medicine, Fenugreek tea is simple to find.

Goldenseal tea is the other indicated tea for tooth infection. Goldenseal is a Turmeric-related herb, and it has much of Turmeric's anti-inflammatory and immune-stimulating properties.

For tooth infection, Goldenseal often has natural antibiotic and antibacterial effects. To cure a tooth infection, consume up to three cups per day.

2. ACNE

As pores get obstructed or contaminated with bacteria, acne grows. In the United States, acne is the most prevalent skin disease, impacting about 80% of people in their lives. Specific home remedies may be used by people to control the oil levels in the skin better, minimize inflammation, destroy bacteria, and avoid possible breakouts in acne.

Acne Traditional Remedies

Any of the more common acne treatments require the use of herbal medicinal extracts, several of which have been utilized for hundreds of years by conventional medicine practitioners.

Below, we speak about the right acne home remedies, what the research suggests, and lifestyle improvements that might improve.

Tea Tree Oil

Tea tree oil is a natural anti-inflammatory and antibacterial agent, which suggests it could destroy P. acnes, the acne-causing bacteria.

The anti-inflammatory effects of tea tree oil indicate that it may also decrease pimples' redness and swelling.

The established evidence for tea tree oil & acne was looked at in a 2015 research article. The researchers observed that tea tree oil products might decrease acne sores in individuals with mild to severe acne.

How to use oil from a tea tree: In creams, gels, and essential oils, individuals may add tea tree oil to their acne. If essential oils are used by humans, they often dilute them first in a carrier oil.

Oil From Jojoba

Jojoba natural, waxy material derived from the seeds of the (shrub) is jojoba oil. Jojoba oil's waxy substances can help fix damaged skin, which implies it may also help accelerate the healing of wounds, including acne lesions.

Some of the jojoba oil compounds can help decrease skin inflammation, which implies that redness and swelling around pimples, whiteheads, and other inflamed lesions can be reduced.

Researchers gave 133 individuals clay face masks that included jojoba oil in a 2012 report. People showed a 54 % improvement in their acne after six weeks of using the masks two to three days per week.

How to make use of jojoba oil: Try blending the essential oil of jojoba with a clay face mask cream or gel and adding it to acne. Otherwise, put on a cotton pad a few drops of jojoba oil and massage this gently across acne sores.

Aloe Vera

Aloe vera is a potent anti-inflammatory and antibacterial medication, which ensures that the presence of acne can be lowered, and acne breakouts can be prevented.

Aloe vera is an excellent moisturizer and includes tones of water, so it is extremely appropriate for people who might get dry skin from several other anti-acne items. In a 2014 report, researchers gave individuals with moderate to mild acne aloe vera gel and tretinoin cream to use for eight weeks, a popular OTC acne treatment.

Compared to individuals who used only tretinoin gel, the researchers showed a substantial improvement both in inflammatory and non-inflammatory acne.

Usage aloe vera gel: Aim to rinse the acne sores and then add at least ten percent aloe vera content to a thin coat of cream or gel.

Honey

For thousands of years, honey is used to cure skin issues, such as acne. It includes several antioxidants that may help to clean clogged pores of waste and debris.

Due to its antibacterial and wound-healing properties, physicians use honey in dressings.

Usage of honey: Rub a little honey into the pimples with a clean finger/cotton pad. Or else, add a face or a body mask of honey.

Garlic

Many practitioners of traditional medicine use garlic to cure illnesses and improve the body's capacity to combat germs and illnesses.

Garlic produces organosulfur compounds that have anti-inflammatory and antibacterial properties that are normal. Organosulfur compounds, which help the

Vintage illustration #3_Garlic

body combat infections, may also help strengthen the immune system.

Usage of garlic: People should incorporate enough garlic to their diet to combat the inflammation and infections induced by acne. Whole garlic cloves are chewed by certain people, spread on toast, or turned into a hot beverage.

Garlic powders or tablets may also be purchased by customers from most supermarkets and natural health outlets.

Green Tea

Green tea includes a category of polyphenol antioxidants named catechins in large concentrations. There is so many sebum, and natural body oils, in the pores of most people with acne but not enough antioxidants. Antioxidants allow the body to break down products that can harm healthy cells from chemicals and waste products. Green tea will help rid any of the debris and waste that has been collected in open sores of acne.

There are also compounds in green tea that can help:
- Reduce sebum development in the skin
- Reduced P. acnes
- Inflammation reduction

Usage of green tea: Green tea can benefit when people drink it or use green tea on their skin, but researchers claim little current evidence. However, after eight weeks of utilizing polyphenol green tea extract, one study discovered a 79% to 89% decrease in whiteheads and blackheads.

Echinacea

Echinacea purpurea can contain compounds that help eliminate bacteria and viruses, including P. acnes, also known as purple coneflower. Many people assume that Echinacea, including colds and flu, will strengthen the immune system and decrease inflammation and then use it to fend off or avoid infections.

How to make use of echinacea: People should add Echinacea-containing creams to places where they have acne lesions or have supplements of Echinacea.

Rosemary

Rosemary extract includes chemicals and substances that have antibacterial, antioxidant, and anti-inflammatory effects or Rosmarinus Officinalis. The impact of rosemary extract on acne has been studied in few reports; however, a 2013 report on mice models and human cells showed that rosemary extract can minimize inflammation from its acne-causing bacteria P. acnes.

Coconut oil

Coconut oil produces anti-inflammatory and antibacterial agents, much as most natural treatments. These properties imply that coconut oil can destroy bacteria that cause acne and reduce pimple redness and swelling. In open acne sores, coconut oil can also accelerate healing.

Basil

According to the Little Barn Apothecary experts, the green herb is much stronger astringent than alcohol. It helps get things out of the skin and works as an antiseptic. It can assist with any irritation that is generally associated with acneic skin and tends to manage oil production, which is a reason for certain breakouts. You should easily mix up a few stems and smear them on the face for a DIY cleaning mask.

Cajeput

Cajeput is identical to a tea tree. it is distilled from the white wood tree bark. It's very useful for inflammatory clearing and astringent properties. Plus, it's antiseptic as well because it helps kill the bacteria that cause breakouts. And, like basil, if you've whiteheads, this herb is the perfect spice.

Lavender

Lavender is all for relaxing, as you've probably guessed. If you've redness, to lower it and relax the skin, you should add lavender. It's amazing for the senses, too; it helps calm.

Chamomile

Another herb that's particularly useful for washing the skin is chamomile. To make a relaxing facial buff, or search for it in the all-natural cleanser. It is recommended to combine it with oatmeal natural and clays.

Rose Oil

Another soothing powerhouse is rose oil, and it appears to be an excellent solution to those frustrating flare-ups. "Scoggins notes," Hormonal acne reacts very well to a rose. In rose oil, that arises from the petals, there is much of balancing, so it is perfect to use for target breakouts.

Geranium

Look for the geranium in the skin-care items if the breakouts are the blackhead type. Geranium oil tends to reduce down the symptoms of aging and manage the intake of oil. That's important because blackheads turn up any time when you've got an overproduction of clogged pores and oil.

Yarrow Blue

In natural form, this exquisite herb isn't as fragile as it seems. Blue yarrow is a very good astringent that helps facilitate the healing of the skin, and it is one of those really antiseptic herbs that extracts infection from the skin and avoids breakouts. For inflamed skin and also blackheads, it is fine. Aim for it while the skin is in freak out mode full-on.

Hibiscus

Switch to a floral stunner like this. Hibiscus has been labeled the Botox of nature. It's also nice to clear the skin and help shore it up. It helps to reduce the presence of wrinkles and fine lines. It's beautiful, but strong, in other words.

Vintage illustration #4_Geranium

3. ALLERGIES

Your effects can be relieved by over-the-counter medications, but certain herbal treatments can also work. Here are a couple of ones to suggest trying.

Butterbur

It is a form of herb that is a natural cure for migraines with a good reputation. And, it has been shown to greatly enhance unpleasant allergy effects in various studies. One study of 125 individuals with hay fever in the British Medical Journal showed that butterbur performed almost like cetirizine, which is known as Zytrec. The researchers have concluded that a butterbur is a clever option for someone who wants to boost their allergy symptoms whilst preventing antihistamines' sedative impact. While cetirizine is deemed a medication for non-sedating allergies, this study showed that subjects who take it exhaustion and drowsiness were encountered.

Garlic

In the homemade tomato sauce, raw garlic is not a must. It is also an essential aspect of every health regime due to its potential to effectively reverse sickness. In addition, garlic is a powerful anti-inflammatory & immune enhancer containing quercetin, which reduces histamine. Quercitin is at the forefront of the list of natural substances that have been proven to enhance symptoms when it comes to treating spring allergies naturally. That's how the histamine levels spike when you're having spring allergies while the body attempts to resist the allergens. It has been shown in studies that garlic not only enhances immune function but also serves as a natural antihistamine with its quercetin. And testing has shown that, in many allergy-fighting drugs and supplements, quercetin (plant-derived) has rapidly become the main component.

Stinging Nettle Leaf

It's a perpetual flowering plant that dates back to ancient Greece and is being used medicinally for centuries. Stinging nettle is already found to have outstanding anti-inflammatory properties with respect to seasonal allergies; furthermore, tests have shown that the stinging nettle bioactive components can potentially inhibit several inflammatory reactions. This is meaningful because it is such inflammatory activities that really cause symptoms of seasonal allergy.

Rosemary

Fresh and dried rosemary are common additives to several culinary creations. The study has shed light on rosemary potential to help combat allergic symptoms and provide asthma sufferers with relief in recent years. According to the study published in the Restorative Medicine Journal, this famous herb includes rosmarinic acid, which has both antioxidant and anti-inflammatory properties, according to the study published in the Restorative Medicine Journal.

The analysis also indicates that rosmarinic acid is the free radical scavenger that might inhibit some white blood cells inflammatory responses and allergic antibodies. In other terms, rosmarinic acid must serve to relieve the effects of seasonal allergies.

Caution: if you have rosmarinic acid as the medication, to reduce possible moderate stomach discomfort, it can help to take it with meals.

Turmeric

A popular spice widely used in Thai, Indian, and other cuisines are turmeric. And there is an endless list of the health benefits of turmeric, according to ongoing research, that brings this tasty spice as effective as plenty of pharmaceuticals, if not more so. Curcumin is turmeric's most effective active compound, and animal experiments have demonstrated that it can substantially mitigate and suppress allergic reactions. Another research of 214 people having allergic rhinitis conducted by the American Allergy, Asthma, and Immunology College showed that those who used curcumin for eight weeks eased their congestion and sneezing and increased nasal ventilation relative to all who took a placebo.

Vintage illustration #6_Tumeric

4. ANXIETY

As a cure for anxiety, many herbal therapies have been tested, but further study is required to clarify the hazards and benefits. This is what we know and do not know:

Kava

Kava proved to be a potential anxiety remedy. However, records of significant liver injury, also for short-term usage, prompted the FDA to provide recommendations on the use of kava-containing dietary supplements. Although these original liver toxicity findings have been disputed, if you are contemplating utilizing items containing kava, use special care and include your specialist in the decision.

Passion Flower

A few limited clinical trials indicate that the passion flower can assist with anxiety. Passion flowers are mixed with other herbs in several consumer items, rendering it hard to discern each plant's distinctive characteristics. When consumed as instructed, passion flower is usually considered healthy, although some reports have shown it can induce drowsiness, dizziness, and misunderstanding.

Valeriana

Individuals that used valerian showed fewer distress and tension in several trials. People have reported no advantages in other trials. Valerian is usually deemed healthy at prescribed levels, although as long-term safety tests are incomplete unless approved by the doctor, do not take it for more than a couple of weeks at a time. Any adverse effects, such as migraine, drowsiness, and dizziness, may be induced.

Chamomile

Research suggests that chamomile is usually deemed healthy for short-term usage and may be effective in decreasing anxiety symptoms. Although, when combined with blood-thinning medications, chamomile may boost the risk of bleeding. Chamomile usage may induce allergic reactions in certain individuals that are susceptible to the chamomile-containing family of plants. Ragweed, daisies, marigolds, & chrysanthemums are additional representatives of this family.

Lavender

Many researches indicate that oral lavender or lavender aromatherapy may decrease anxiety, although there is minimal and tentative research. Oral lavender can induce headaches and constipation. Appetite can also improve, the sedative impact of some drugs and supplements can improve, and low blood pressure can be induced.

Lemon Balm

Preliminary evidence suggests that certain signs of anxiety, including nervousness and excitability, may be minimized by a lemon balm. Lemon balm is normally well-tolerated for short-term usage and is deemed healthy but may induce nausea and stomach pain. The FDA is not regulating herbal products in the same way drugs do. The consistency of certain supplements can still be a concern, considering improved quality management legislation in force since 2010. Bear in mind; natural does not necessarily mean safety.

5. ASTHMA

You probably do realize that pharmaceutical medications are the greatest medical expense due to asthma, whether you have asthma or care about someone who does. In the United States, asthma medication costs $6 billion a year, according to the ALA (American Lung Association).

Keeping track of multiple inhalers and drugs may also be a pain, in addition to the cost of asthma medicines. You may be worried about finding a herbal cure or complementary therapy for your asthma, whether you are seeking more natural means of asthma treatment or searching for strategies to improve the management of your asthma symptoms. A variety of individuals with asthma are exploring alternative therapy to strengthen their asthma symptom regulation. Most people use alternative medicines, especially for allergic diseases. In reality, as many as 40 % of people with an allergic condition are seeking a natural cure.

As natural cures for asthma, a variety of herbs have been reported, but it is recommended that before trying these asthma medications, people should be vigilant.

These potential care methods and the dangers and advantages involved with them include:

Garlic

Thanks to its anti-inflammatory effects, garlic is used as a natural remedy to treat many illnesses, particularly heart disease. It may make sense that garlic can often help alleviate asthma symptoms because asthma is an inflammatory condition. However, it is stated that there have not been any experimental studies examining the impact of garlic on symptoms of asthma. Hence, its function is unclear in the treatment of asthma. However, the usage of garlic as an additional option for asthma is being investigated at present.

Tussilago Farfara (Coltsfoot)

As a cough suppressant, it's been used medicinally. In ancient times, the plant was used to cure lung problems such as asthma and also various coughs by smoking.

Ginkgo Biloba

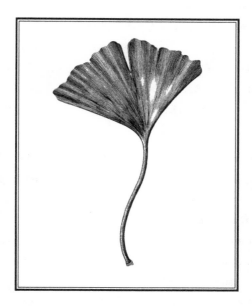

There is a large variety of indications for ginkgo, one of the earliest herbs in usage today. Ginkgo acts to suppress (platelet-activating factor PAF), a potent platelet aggregator inducer, and anaphylactic reactions in asthma sufferers.

For the cure of asthma, thrombosis, allergic reactions, and shock, natural herbs that promote anti-PAF behavior are considered to aid. One analysis found that a 600 mg standardized dosage of ginkgo in patients with asthma decreased airway hypersensitivity.

Curcuma Longa (Turmeric)

Turmeric is a part of the ginger family which has been used for centuries as a coloring agent, medication, and spice. Diarylhepanoids, curcumin, found in the vibrantly yellow rhizome, is the active constituents. In an unregulated analysis in India, 60% of asthma patients treated with 6-12 g of turmeric powder fried in ghee reported relief from their symptoms. In both acute or chronic conditions, curcumin is an effective anti-inflammatory, and it is known to act to minimize inflammation in a number of biological pathways. Curcumin had comparable effectiveness to cortisone and phenylbutazone in certain models tested.

Scutellaria Baicalensis (Chinese Skullcap)

In TCM (traditional Chinese medicine), this plant's roots are used for a range of illnesses, including asthma. The Chinese skullcap includes flavone derivatives that prevent histamine release from the mast cells in vitro, including wogonin, baicalin, and baicalein. In asthmatic guinea pigs' independent tracheal muscle, baicalin displayed antiasthmatic activity (anticholinergic and antihistaminic activity). The treatment of asthma needs to reduce hypersensitivity and inflammation in the airways.

Grindeliaspp (Grindelia)

This is a bronchospasmolytic expectorant herb. In the management of spasmodic respiratory diseases such as asthma and bronchitis, it is traditionally prescribed. The basic indication is described in the 1983 British Herbal Pharmacopoeia as asthma (bronchial) with tachycardia. In addition to skin diseases, Native Americans utilized grindelia for bronchial problems, where grindelia gradually attracted Catholic missionaries' interest. In the U.S. Pharmacopoeia 1882–1926, the grindelia flowering tops and dried leaf were official and were in the National Form, 1926–1960.

Echinacea And Licorice Root

One research investigating the usage of a variety of various herbs to cure asthma showed that not only was Echinacea, a herb sometimes used to cure upper respiratory infections unsuccessful, but a variety of side effects were also correlated with it. The complications associated with Echinacea usage are worsening asthma, skin rashes and potential liver damage if taken with the other medicines. Likewise, as a potential remedy for asthma, licorice root, which has antioxidant and anti-inflammatory properties and is often used by people who have asthma to soothe their lungs, was discovered to be unsuccessful and often correlated with adverse effects such as increased blood pressure. It is stated that no clinical studies have proven that both Echinacea or licorice root is an effective therapy for asthma and that there have been several indications that in certain people, Echinacea may worsen symptoms of asthma.

Ginger

Ginger is often believed to alleviate inflammation, and a new report has found that oral ginger extracts are correlated with improving the symptoms of asthma. However, the research did not demonstrate that ginger's use contributed to any real lung function change. Consequently, it is cautioned about utilizing this research as an experimental therapy for asthma to draw some assumptions regarding ginger usage. Additional experiments are also being performed to more thoroughly determine whether or not ginger will better manage the effects of asthma.

Adhatoda Vasica (Adhatoda)

In India and South East Asia, this herb is a tiny evergreen shrub that's located at lower altitudes. For decades, the leaf was used to combat asthma, where it serves as a bronchodilator as well as a moderate expectorant. In order to aid with expectoration, Adhatoda often acts by decreasing mucous viscosity. The quinazoline alkaloids (0.5 to 2%) are essential constituents of the adhatoda root. The key alkaloid is 45-95 percent vasicine and is the initial cause of the medication bromhexine, which is now used to help in expectoration.

6. BREATH

The EPA revealed that every day we take from 17,280 - 23,040 breaths. We want each one of those to smell nice.

Common causes of bad breath:

1. Gingivitis: Due to the accumulation of plaque and degradation between the teeth, this significant smelly breath source happens. If you let it go, it will lead to missing teeth and extreme infections. You require specialized dental care to go with your herbal remedies when your halitosis is followed by deep purple gums, inflammation, bleeding, and painful brushing.

2. Cavities : Overtime of anaerobic bacteria can occupy a cavity. Such germs will produce a foul scent in the mouth. This often involves a doctor, and if overlooked, it can transform into a life-endangered infection.

3. Dry Mouth : Stinky breath often occurs from benign reasons, including dry mouth. If you snore, breathe with open mouth, speak a lot, etc., your mouth will dry out.

Peppermint

Peppermint flavoring is used in several kinds of toothpaste, and this is not by chance. It has the power to offer a new, clean feeling to the mouth. Peppermint essential oils (real peppermint, not flavoring) do a lot more than produce a fresh feeling. One research found that peppermint oils help more efficiently mitigate bad breath than a chemical rinse developed by a laboratory.

Tea Tree

Among natural health experts, tea tree oil has been recognized for its toxicity to unhealthy things that cause bad breath. With these strong properties, the tea tree oil extract effectiveness in mouth rinses has been investigated by researchers. One such analysis showed that a broader variety of microorganisms were eliminated by tea tree oil in comparison to the chemical chlorhexidine. Another analysis showed that a halitosis-associated bacterium, Solobacterium moorei, was particularly susceptible to the tea tree oil effects. Used in a rinse, in the war against bad breath, it provides a total cleaning effect. Tea tree oil, which may induce bad breath, has also been found effective in treating Candida.

Sage

The Sage has been regarded as a medicinal herb since ancient times. Modern study has validated its potency only against harmful organisms and its effective ability to combat halitosis. Sage has been shown to be successful against organisms including Candida albicans, Porphyromonas gingivalis, and Streptococcus mutans, that cause bad breath.

Myrrh

It has been used in a multitude of forms for centuries. Myrrh is an effective natural cure for those trying to combat bad breath, whatever the source since it aids cleanse the mouth from germs and often treats problems that could promote further development.

Clove

Poor breath is deemed a product of Qi stagnation in Chinese medicine. Clove fosters Qi flow and clove has a history of remedying bad breath in Chinese medicine. Clove has been described as an important part of mouth rinses in modern studies. In one research, in terms of flavor, after-taste and ease of usage, participants preferred this to a chemical-based mouth rinse. Mouth rinses utilizing herbs such as cloves often offered suitable options for people who were unwilling to use chemical cleaners.

Needle Of Pine

For a variety of medical remedies, pine resins and oils have traditionally been used. Naturally, pine produces terpene alcohols that are active cleansing agents and toxic to damaging organisms. Pine oils have also been determined by researchers to give strong antioxidant properties. The pine needle, as part of the mouth rinse, encourages good mouth health.

Eucalyptus

Eucalyptus has shown impressive efficacy in lowering bad breath. In a 2010 report, by substantially decreasing volatile sulfur compounds (that render your breath wretched), eucalyptus was observed to remove mouth malodor. The effectiveness of eucalyptus in research has shown that its cleansing properties have been successful both in the laboratory and in nature.

Ginger And Mango
Prepare the rhizomes of decoction. Gargle twice a day with it.

Cubeb
Grab a glass of water that is slightly wet. Add five drops of the oil from Cubeb. Swish it twice or three times a day.
Or make the Cubeb infusion. With it, swish.

Lemon Balm
Chew out the Lemon Balm leaves and stem.

Guava (Amrood)
Have a leaf decoction prepared, then swish with it.

Dill
Chew half a tablespoon of the seeds of dill.
OR: Make a tea with dill leaves. Drink twice.

RECEPIE

Chop leaves of Parsley. Adding water with four Cloves in it. Simmer. Using it as a cleaner for your mouth.

Take 1 tsp of Carom (Ajwain) and 4 teaspoons of Laung (Clove). Boil the water in a cup. Cool. Swish twice a day with this water.

Gargle with 1 tsp of Honey and Cinnamon in the morning.

Using a combination of Solanum Xanthocarpum and some vinegar as a combination.

1/4 cup of Solanum Xanthocarpum juice, combine 1-2 tbsp of vinegar. Twice a day as a mouthwash.

Dip a few pieces of Asafoetida (Hing) in 1/2 a bowl of water with 2-3 cloves.

Only leaving it overnight. To prevent bad breath, gargle every day.

To prevent bad breath, gargle with this water

---

7. BACK PAIN

To soothe your back, there is a large range of herbal treatments that can either minimize drug consumption or offer additional value to current medical care.

THE FOUNDATION OF AMERICAN PAIN OFTEN LISTS THESE HERBS:

Boswellia and Willow Bark for pain relief
Ginseng for fibromyalgia
Kava for migraine with tension and neuropathic discomfort
St. John's Wort for sciatica, inflammation, and neuropathic suffering from
Valerian root for spasms & muscle cramps
White willow bark, Devil's claw, and Cayenne can decrease back pain

---

Every Day, Consume An Anti-Inflammatory Drink

Several antioxidants, anti-inflammatory, and even anti-cancer agents might build up in the blood as you consistently eat anti-inflammatory foods. Over a duration of time, such potent agents can play a major role in decreasing and preventing inflammatory reactions in the body.

It can help minimize your back pain to consume these nutritious beverages regularly.

1. Golden Milk

There are antioxidant, anti-arthritic, and anti-inflammatory effects of Turmeric, an Asian spice. Mixing a tiny amount (1/2 tsp) of turmeric powder in a cup of warm milk is a simple way to consume Turmeric. If you want a sweet flavor, you should add honey/stevia to the milk. Ideally, have this drink before bedtime to enable the anti-inflammatory mechanism to function when you are asleep.

In certain individuals, eating dairy products can raise inflammation. In those situations, it may be helpful to try plant-based milk, like almond milk.

2. Tart Cherry Juice

Cherries are high in antioxidants and anti-inflammatory drugs. Cherry juice may help alleviate chronic or exercise-induced body pain. Cherry juice is widely accessible for purchase in food stores and includes the tart cherry extract. Try to consume a cup of cherry juice on a normal basis and see whether it has a beneficial impact on back pain recovery.

3. Green Tea With Ginger

Ginger-green tea packets can be ordered from convenience stores, and you can comfortably enjoy a cup at work or at home. You can also try suffused-herbal beverages, like ginger-green tea, which provides both green tea and ginger's pain-relieving properties. Such anti-inflammatory agents will build up in your body over time but having these beverages in your everyday diet can help decrease total inflammation and stop fresh inflammatory pain.

8. BITES AND STINGS

Summer is here in all its beauty, and that suggests more time spent outdoors for many of us. Like every gardener or outdoor lover acknowledges, once you have an unfortunate experience with insect bites or stings, it's usually only a matter of time. The impact may vary from mild pain to infections or even disease. Mosquitos, ticks, black flies, fleas, bees, horse flies, chiggers & deer flies are some of the most popular biting or stinging pests.

A great alternative to insecticide, which also includes additives such as DEET and permethrin that may have harmful consequences on many, can be natural remedies. As the phrase goes, "An ounce of protection is worth a pound of treatment," and when it comes to insect bites, this is no less real. For their insect-repellent effects, several essential oils (plants) are valuable. Pennyroyal, citronella, cedar-wood, cinnamon leaf oil, eucalyptus, & catnip oil are a couple of the most popular. For making a bug spray, these may be applied to water. Notice that pregnant women should stop Pennyroyal. Alternatively, there are widely distributed citronella candles.

The main objectives are calming pain and curing the skin if you try your utmost to hold pests at bay, but sometimes wind up with a sting or bite. In this case, the following herbs could be beneficial.

Plantago Major (Plantain)

For insect bites, fresh plantain leaves may be used. New plantain leaves may be combined with bentonite clay and water to form a paste to produce a poultice. Alternatively, it is possible to chew a leaf and position it right over the bite.

Calendula Officinalis (Calendula)

Calendula oil and fresh leaves may soothe skin irritated, itchy, and can ensure effective bite and sting healing. With calendula, beeswax, & antiseptic essential oils, like rosemary, tea tree, and lavender, a basic salve may be produced.

Symphytum Officinale (Comfrey)

For multiple skin disorders, including rashes, scrapes, and injuries, Comfrey enriched oil or fresh juice through leaves may be used topically. It can alleviate scratching and discomfort due to bites and stings.

Hamamelis (Witch Hazel)

Witch hazel distillate is readily available in supermarkets, and for mild skin irritations, it is an over-the-counter relief. Integrate three parts of baking soda to 1.5 parts of witch hazel to make an itch-soothing potion.

These medicines are created from herbs & ingredients that are readily found. A few (or all) on hand is prudent, particularly in the summer months, when bites, stings, scratches, and scrapes eventually occur.

Mentha Piperita (Peppermint)

Cooling peppermint oil and crushed leaves may soothe itchy or swollen bites.

9. BRONCHITIS, PNEUMONIA, AND CHEST COLD

Most of us got a typical cough. However, it occurs in a respiratory condition known as bronchitis because this simple cough is followed by serious symptoms such as breathlessness & phlegm. A cough or flu further compromises the immune function, and people are then at a greater risk of contracting bronchitis. If not managed, persistent bronchitis will progress to asthma and chronic obstructive pulmonary disease (COPD), which may be life-threatening. Bronchitis may also be divided into acute or recurrent, much like any other disease. Inflammation or swelling of the bronchial tubes that hold oxygen between the lung, mouth, and nose. Those dealing with bronchitis find it very hard to inhale oxygen into the lungs. A frequent source of bronchitis is inhaling toxic fumes and air that includes pollen. For certain people who are dealing with bronchitis, inhaling toxic air may be worse.

In reality, smoking is believed to be the primary cause of bronchitis, and smokers are at a greater risk of contracting this disease. This is because cigarettes produce numerous chemicals, and the surface of the bronchial tube or surface is irritated as people inhale these chemicals. This is why they get recurrent bronchitis. Smoking induces cells to create more mucus than usual, allowing the bronchial tubes to become inflamed. This mucus also has the potential to cover the whole lining of bronchi, contributing to the buildup of bronchitis-causing harmful bacteria. This worsens the bronchitis state of the person suffering. Symptoms of bronchitis include phlegm or dry cough, fever, shortness of breath, and fatigue too.

Saunth (Dry Ginger), Pipli (Long Pepper), and Kali Mirchi (Black Pepper)

In the event of enlarged bronchial passages, Saunth has anti-inflammatory effects that offer relief. To aid in getting rid of nose congestion, Kali mirch is really helpful. Long pepper, or pipli, is well recognized for its anti-inflammatory effects. For immediate results, Ayurveda specialist B.N. Sinha recommends combining all three ingredients in powdered shape, along with honey and drinking the mixture three times a day.

Giloy Juice

Giloy (Tinospora Cordifolia) is a herb of Ayurveda derivation that was used and refreshed for centuries in the medicine of Indian. Giloy has a reassuring encouragement on the throat lining and thereby allows the inflamed bronchial lining to offer relief. Drink the juice for relaxation once in the morning and once in the evening per day.

Trikatu And Garlic Powder

It is recommended to produce a mixture of four parts of garlic powder and one part of trikatu, including a little honey, and taking it twice a day. Although garlic in any kitchen is a popular ingredient, it was highly prized in ancient times for its various health-beneficial properties that are still followed today in many cultures.

Soup Of Ginger

Ginger, particularly in Ayurveda healing, has different advantages. Ginger has characteristics that are really useful in cough care. If it's not ginger soup, you can drink ginger tea, which is just as effective. The ginger powder, which is ground, is derived from the root of ginger. It is a small off-white substance with a heavy fragrance and a pungent taste, or somewhat brownish.

Massage Of Mustard Oil

Mustard oil is derived from the seeds of mustard (black, white, and brown) and is brown/amber reddish. Since ancient times, it has been widely used in east and north India and comes with a bevy of beneficial effects.

A soft mustard oil massage tends to offer relaxation against a sore chest. The congestion in the lungs is relieved by massaging with mustard oil.

It is recommended that people suffering from bronchitis, apart from these basic and quick to reach home remedies, to avoid curd & other cold items that could aggravate the disease. Keep warm, particularly during the winter months, when people are more vulnerable to cold and cough bouts. If one is prone to cough and cold allergies, smoking must be stopped.

10. SUNBURNS AND BURNS

Sometimes sunburns happen, even among the most conscientious of wearers of sunscreen. Fortunately, there are a number of different approaches to treat a burn at home, utilizing ingredients that you might already have on your bathroom shelves or in your refrigerator.

Plantain

One of the most common folk remedies in North America used for the treatment of burns is Plantain (Plantago major). For a relaxing effect, plant juice is added directly to the mild burns. It is effective in the management of bug bites as well. It's antibacterial, like comfrey, includes allantoin, a phytochemical anti-inflammatory that speeds the healing of wounds and encourages the development of fresh skin cells.

Aloe Vera

Aloe vera gel alleviates discomfort and inflammation as well as speeds the mechanism of recovery. Aloe has been in use since ancient times, and the efficacy of this natural medicinal treatment for treating wounds, including frostbite and burns induced by radiation therapy, has been supported by modern science. Aloe includes carboxypeptidase and bradykinesia enzymes, which mitigate discomfort, decrease inflammation, and minimize redness and swelling. It also has important antifungal and antibacterial properties that lead to infection prevention. It is possible to use either aloe gel bought in the shop or fresh juice from an aloe farm. As an integral part of a personal first-aid package, often, people held a live aloe plant.

Gotu Kola

In Ayurvedic medicine, Gotu Kola (Centella Asiatica) is strongly appreciated for its skin rejuvenating capacity. It can speed up the process of healing and help to avoid scarring. Taken internally, when used with Vit C, it stimulates the synthesis of collagen, an essential skin repair component. Mix equal sections of the Gotu kola powder and aloe gel for a successful topical herbal remedy for mild burns or sunburn.

Oregon Grape

Mahonia aquifolium (Oregon Grape) may be very effective in the treatment of burns since it includes berberine, which has been shown to defend against viruses, bacteria, and fungi.

Scientific evidence has shown that berberine-containing plants activate the immune system and combat infection. A potent antioxidant, Oregon Grape root, produces tannins that relieve skin inflammation, discomfort, and scratching.

Comfrey's

In Chinese Traditional Medicine, Comfrey (Symphytum Officinale) was used for more than 2000 years. As an ointment or poultice applied as a natural cure for burns, sprains, fractured bones as well as other wounds, one of the most common applications of comfrey leaves is to facilitate quick healing of all skin lesions and bone breaks.

Calendula

Calendula officinalis, also known as marigold, has a long tradition of usage to remedy burns and other skin inflammation.

Calendula is known to have antiseptic andanti-inflammatory properties that stimulate the development of outer skin cells and help facilitate healing. For acute radiotherapy dermatitis, moderate skin burns, scalds, shaving burns, moderate sunburn, and windburn even, calendula can be used. It acts to eliminate blisters and scar tissue instantly and efficiently. It can also be used as an eyewash in the circumstance of some chemical burn. When it's used as a compress added to the burn region, calendula is the most effective. Notice that calendula, along with ragweed, is a part of the composite family, which can result in allergic reactions.

Slippery Elm (Ulmus Rubra)

It has been used as a medicinal remedy for burns, cuts, boils, ulcers, and different skin inflammations by Native Americans for decades. Slippery Elm is a demulcent, diuretic, and anti-inflammatory mucilaginous agent that can be used as a topical remedy for inflammatory skin problems.

Burns Healing Internal Formula

By use of vulnerary herbs for extreme burns can aid speed healing and decrease scarring. Symphytum officinale is a long-standing curing agent, so Calendula officinalis facilitates dermal circulation and strengthens connective tissue development in the basement membrane. The study is minimal; however, it is suspected that Calendula officinalis promotes wound healing by facilitating glycoprotein & collagen production, hastening regeneration of dermis. Hypericum perforatum tends to decrease pain and repair nerve ends that are damaged. Centella asiatica has been shown to be useful in supporting post-burn epithelial regeneration.

You may prepare this formula as a tincture or even a tea.
- Centella Asiatica
- Symphytum Officinale
- Calendula Officinalis
- Hypericum Perforatum

Blend in similar proportions. For a week or more, take 1 tsp of the blended tincture six times every day. Using 1/2 ounce of each herb to create the mix to prepare it as a drink. Each cup of hot water and strain, steep 1 tbsp of the herb mixture. If necessary, drink five to six cups a day, and proceed for one week or two.

Lavender

The pure essential oil of lavender (Lavandula Angustifolia) is considered one of the leading cures for burns by many aromatherapists.

It's antiseptic and analgesic and, without dilution, is the essential oil that can be added to the skin directly.

It stops infection, lowers inflammation, facilitates regeneration and inhibits, or eliminates scar tissue development.

As indicated by the numerous lavender-scented baby items on the market, it is deemed the best oil to use with kids.

The lavender scent often has healing effects, relaxing the nerves following injuries.

Vintage illustration #11_Lavender

11. CONSTIPATION

Constipation is described as passing or getting less than three bowel movements per week by stiff, dry stool. Constipation, one of the most prevalent intestinal complaints, affects most individuals at any stage in their lives.

Some individuals develop short-term constipation related to sudden adjustments in lifestyle, stress, travel, or surgery, whereas others have permanent (persistent for many weeks or longer) constipation. If you have persistent constipation, you undoubtedly recognize how your life's quality will be greatly impacted by it.

It is more frequent in women and in people over the age of 65. While constipation can impact anybody, it also appears to arise during pregnancy or after delivery and can be the product of an underlying disorder or side effect of drugs (like opioid pain medication).

STIMULANT LAXATIVES
Cascara Sagrada
Aloe
Rhubarb
Senna Tea
Senna
Buckthorn

Stimulant laxatives, also called anthraquinone laxatives, are many natural laxatives and "dieter's teas."

Any of these herbs, including senna, are licensed as over-the-counter constipation therapies. In fact, people can become reliant on them and use them for weeks, months, and years at a time in an attempt to get a normal bowel movement, while they are intended for being short-term treatments.

Before using herbal laxatives, it is essential to speak with the primary care physician, and they cannot be taken for more than a week because they are under medical supervision.

Prolonged usage can cause the bowels to lose the freedom to navigate independently and has been correlated with persistent diarrhea, liver toxicity, muscle weakness, potassium deficiency, cardiac function disorders, anf failure of the kidney or liver.

It is painful and may cause life unpleasant. You want instant relief when you are feeling weighed down and bloated. To ease constipation, you might be willing to use herbal cures.

Constipation is described as having less than three weekly bowel movements. It can be recurrent, or it can occur rarely. Certain signs include:
• Hard stuffed stools
• Exertion to do a bowel movement
• Feeling as if you're "blocked" or will not empty your intestines
• The need for assistance to empty your rectum
• Pain in the abdomen
• Nausea, puffiness

Seeking herbal remedies against constipation is fairly simple. In reality, several laxatives that are over the counter contain herbal ingredients. Anthraquinones, or compounds that have a stimulant impact on the intestines are found in most laxative herbs. By pulling fluid into the colon and growing peristalsis, these laxatives perform. Peristalsis is the intestine contraction, helping to transfer fluid to the rectum from the colon. When constipated, incorporating fiber and fluids is necessary.

Buckthorn (Cascara Sagrada)
This is a common herbal laxative which comes from a species of the buckthorn tree's bark extract. This extract functions by enough irritating the colon to facilitate bowel movements. Short-term usage is normally well accepted, although stomach discomfort or electrolyte deficiency can be induced. Long-term usage can lead to liver injuries varying from moderate to serious liver failure.

Psyllium

A part of the genus of plantain plants, psyllium, is the laxative of natural fiber that helps generate bulk stools. For the prevention of persistent constipation, psyllium is sometimes used and can be paired with other natural and synthetic laxatives. Such side effects can be induced by it, like:

- Allergic Reaction
- Tiredness and nausea
- Pain in the stomach
- Vomiting

Rhubarb

Although this vegetable may be better regarded as the pie ingredient, it is often used to cure constipation. Rhubarb has a laxative benefit, but because of its tannin material, a report reported in the Ethnopharmacology Journal showed that it often has an antidiarrheal impact. As a consequence, rhubarb can be used for constipation only on a low-term basis.

Senna

It is used prior to some surgical treatments to relieve constipation and clear the intestines. It is assumed that the fruit is gentler than that of the leaf. It can, however, be used only in the low term and also at the prescribed doses. Senna pills are powerful against constipation, and most pharmacy stores will offer them. It has been documented that long-term and high-dose usage induces liver harm.

Slippery Elm

There is a history of this herb being used for constipation. In the GI tract, it activates nerves, which contributes to mucus development and offers relief from constipation. Slippery Elm produces mucilage, a sticky material that covers the GI tract. As a consequence, if administered at the same time, it could limit the absorption of certain drugs.

12. COUGH

There are various forms of cough that have different causes, so it can be helpful to find out the kind of cough people have so that people know which remedy works best.

Dry coughs and tickly coughs are commonly triggered in the back of the mouth by dryness or irritation, so it is a safe idea to get something that can soothe the throat. External causes like allergy, dust, smoke, as well as conditions such as asthma, may also cause them. Chesty coughs are triggered by extra mucus, so it would be beneficial with something that will remove, reduce, or slim this mucus. Colds, flu and other upper respiratory illnesses also follow certain forms of cough.

Pine

Pine is a great herb for relieving coughs.
Bronchosan cough syrup includes pine to help alleviate dry and aggravated coughs, along with honey.

Thyme

Thyme has been used for a long time to treat all sorts of illnesses as an herbal plant, although it is especially effective for respiratory disorders such as cough. It is widely used in the form of tea but, along with other valuable herbs like ivy, star anise oil, and eucalyptus oil, it is also found in the Bronchoforce cure. These ingredients together help loosen and reduce mucus, rendering this a great cure for chesty coughs.

Marshmallow Root

It is a plant used to remedy coughs and sore throats with a long tradition of use. Due to its strong mucilage content, the herb may relieve discomfort arising from coughing. A dense, gluey material that covers the throat is mucilage.
One small research showed that coupled with thyme and ivy, a herbal cough syrup, including marshmallow root, successfully cured coughs arising from the common colds and infections of the respiratory tract. Ninety percent of the participants graded their efficacy as good or really good after twelve days of having the syrup. Often available as the dried herb/bagged tea is the marshmallow root.

Either apply hot water to it and drink it then instantly or first allow it to cool. The more the core of the marshmallow steeps inside water, the more mucilage in the drink would be.

Side effects may involve an upset stomach, although by consuming more water, it could be able to counter this.

Slippery Elm

In order to cure coughing and stomach disorders, Native Americans historically utilized Slippery Elm bark. As it includes a large amount of mucilage, which tends to soothe the cough and sore throat, Slippery Elm is comparable to the marshmallow root. Add dried herb one teaspoon to a cup of warm water to create Slippery Elm tea. Steep for 10 minutes prior to alcohol, at least. It is important to note that the absorption of the medication may interfere with the Slippery Elm.

Mullein

This herb has calming properties and has been widely used since ancient Greece to relieve coughs and inflammation

Lemon And Honey

This home remedy, traditionally used to alleviate a sore throat, is especially beneficial for rough, tickly coughs. The sticky, thick honey really soothes the throat and helps to leave behind a defensive coat.

Vintage illustration #12_Lemon

13. DEPRESSION

To help them control their illness and feel healthier, certain persons with depression choose non-drug interventions. For milder symptoms of depression, natural therapies, and herbal remedies can be good.

Depression is a chronic mood condition with signs varying from moderate to crippling and likely life-threatening.

Saffron

It is a spice that comes from a dried part of a crocus in the iris' family, a herb. According to a report in Alternative Medicine, it successfully manages mild to moderate depression by taking saffron stigma.

Natural food retailers can advertise herbs and supplements as being able to relieve depression. However, some of these approaches have not been proven to be successful in managing depression, according to a study reported in BJPsych Advances.

HERBS TO RELIEVE DEPRESSION

Crataegus Oxyacantha (Hawthorn)
Ginkgo Biloba
Eschscholzia Californica (California Poppy)
Lavandula Angustifolia (Lavender)
Melissa Officinalis (Lemon Balm)
Matricaria Recutita (Chamomile)
Passiflora Incarnate (Maypop, or Purple Passionflower)
Valeriana Officinalis (Valerian)
Piper Methysticum (Kava)

---

14. DIARRHEA

Diarrhea is caused more often than not by slight bouts of food-borne disease or food poisoning. Often, certain viruses can cause moderate diarrhea.

Other diarrhea sources involve consuming so much food, such as fresh fruit, eating things that you are resistant to or intolerant to, such as milk products, or developing gastrointestinal problems, like colitis and irritable bowel syndrome.

If the large intestine and colon require food waste to flow easily, it does not retain moisture and nutrients. The colon will often also take water from the body to enable it to get rid of excess feces in a rush. Either will leave them dehydrated & with important nutrients missing.

Astringent Herbs

Astringent herbs like blackberry leaf or raspberry leaf help to "dry up" the intestinal mucous membranes. Using one heaping tsp, each cup. Drink around half a cup every hour. During pregnancy, there is some debate about using these teas.

Carob powder may be disintegrated into a commercial replenishing drink (hydrating electrolyte), which is rich in fiber. Until guided to do so by the doctor, Do not offer a carob to children.

Bilberry Extract

Vaccinum myrtillus has the astringent characteristic, too. If one take anticoagulants (blood thinners), do not use bilberry. Bilberry may also theoretically connect for drugs for diabetes.

Agrimony is a traditional diarrhea treatment. Agrimony can have a thinning impact on your blood and may increase your blood pressure. If you are dealing with these health problems, talk to your doctor before taking agricultural medicine.

Inflammation Reducers

A plant-based flavonoid, Quercetin, can help reduce inflammation.

Chamomile (Matricaria recutita) is typically taken as a tea. People who are allergic to ragweed, chamomile can interact with hormone drugs and can cause reactions. You should take marshmallow root (Althea officinalis) as a cold-water drink. Just absorb some Root overnight in 1 quart of water Strain. Drink the mixture throughout the day. Marshmallow can interact with some medications, like lithium, that are taken by mouth. The intestines can be soothed by Ulmus fulva (slippery elm powder) or Althaea officinalis (marshmallow root powder). With the powder & a smaller amount, make a paste. Add in the remainder of the water gradually & then simmer down to one pint. Slippery elm has a popular reputation for promoting miscarriage. It can mess with some drugs.

Infection Fighters

Berberine-containing plants can assist in treating infectious diarrhea. This includes barberry (Berberis vulgaris), Hydrastis canadensis (goldenseal), & Berberis aquifolium (Oregon grape). If you are pregnant or nursing, you should NOT take Berberine. If you are on some prescribed medications, consult with the doctor first.

Bulk-Forming Agent

Psyllium can help treat diarrhea, a soluble fiber that came from the husks of seeds of Plantago ovata. It's a bulk-forming agent which tends to firm feces, sucking up water in the colon. For a high volume of water, taking psyllium. Until psyllium is taken, patients with inflammatory bowel disease should appeal to their physicians. Be mindful that while doctors can aid with diarrhea with fiber agents such as psyllium, they are most widely used to treat constipation as a laxative. Before using psyllium for curing diarrhea, talk to your doctor.

Homeopathy

Some research shows that diarrhea may be aided by homeopathic care. In one research, children with severe diarrhea who obtained five days of individualized homeopathic therapy had slightly less time-consuming diarrhea than children who received a placebo. Homeopaths consider the constitutional form of an individual when administering a cure, including the physical, emotional, and intellectual makeup.

When deciding the most effective treatment for a single person, an experienced homeopath considers all of these considerations. Any of the homeopathic treatments that are more successful include:

Arsenicum Album. For foul-smelling diarrhea and burning sensations in the belly and around the anus through food poisoning/diarrhea. This treatment is most suitable for exhausted and restless people and whose symptoms appear to intensify in the cold and progress with warmth. Vomiting can also occur. To avoid diarrhea while traveling, you can also use Arsenicum.

Chamomilla. With a frothy greenish poop that odor like rotten eggs. Used for children specifically, especially those who are argumentative, irritable, and difficult to console. Physicians widely prescribe chamomile for colicky or teething babies.

Calcarea Carbonica. For adolescents who are scared to be isolated or in the dark and who perspire excessively when asleep. Stools may have a sour scent.

Mercurius. Used for foul-smelling diarrhea, which might include blood stains followed by an incomplete emptying sensation. For people who appear to feel tired after bowel motions, undergo drastic shifts in body temperature, perspire excessively, and have a thirst for cool drinks, this treatment is most suitable.

Podophyllum. For gushing, explosive, painless diarrhea, which becomes worse after drinking or eating. Sometimes, fatigue accompanies bowel motions. In the lower extremities, the person for whom this treatment is suitable can suffer painful cramps. For diarrhea suffered from teething, practitioners can use podophyllum in babies.

Sulfur. For irritable, weepy adolescents. With the odor of rotting eggs, they can have diarrhea and a red ring across the anus.

Veratrum Album. For stomach cramps, exhaustion, bloated abdomen, vomiting, chills, profuse and watery diarrhea. The diarrhea is intensified by fruit, and the patient craves cool fluids.

15. FEVER

To cure fever, people often use herbal medicines.

Moringa
Moringa is indeed a tropical plant with a variety of uses in terms of diet and medicine. Vitamins, nutrients, antibacterial agents, and antioxidants are present in almost all areas of the plant. A 2014 research by Trusted Source showed that moringa bark decreased fevers in rabbits.

A few evidences show that it could be gentler against the liver than other medications such as acetaminophen.

Do not use moringa when you are in pregnancy.

Intake of moringa leaves contributes to an unusual skin and mucous membranes condition named Stevens-Johnson syndrome (SJS) from one case study. It means that individuals at risk of having SJS should stop the usage of moringa. It's the first recorded occurrence, though, and the reaction can be regarded to be very unusual.

Kudzu Root
The root of kudzu is indeed an herb that has been used in Chinese traditional medicine. That has an anti-inflammatory effect and can lead to pain relief. A 2012 research also indicates that it decreased fevers in rats, but the trials are required in humans.

Stop using kudzu root when you are:
- Taking tamoxifen
- Hormonally sensitive cancer, like breast cancer
- Taking Rasuvo Take Rasuvo (methotrexate)

Consult to the doctor if you are taking diabetic medicine before you start kudzu root. It can result in low blood sugar, requiring a medicine change.

Diaphoretic Herbs
There is a word called diaphoretic in herbalism. When an herb has such a diaphoretic activity, it indicates that the herb promotes sweating. They get it by enhancing the skin's excretory glands and their impact, which can be stimulating.

They are working, keeping the removal pathways open, facilitating blood supply through the bloodstream, and eliminating the toxins that develop as the body reacts to infection.

The added value of utilizing herbs as the medication is that it is possible to adapt variations to meet the patient's particular situation and terrain. Meadowsweet (Filipendula ulmaria) Herbs like catnip (Nepeta cataria), yarrow (Achillea mille-folium), elderflower (Sambucus nigra), lime blossom (Tilia spp), including pep-permint (Mentha piperita) are widely used for diaphoretics.

16. HEARTBURN, REFLUX AND GERD

Nobody enjoys the sensation, and all of us have known it. The heavy, burning acid slowly creeping up the neck, putting pressure on the chest. Yet it becomes extremely irritating, affecting the lifestyle of those who struggle with GERD (gastroesophageal reflux disease).

But before you rush to the nearest medical store, there are GERD natural remedies you may attempt to relieve the unwelcome side effects of this unpleasant problem.

Peppermint Oil

The leaves of tea contain peppermint oil. Peppermint, though, was traditionally used in the treatment of:

- Headaches
- Colds
- Indigestibility
- Stomach disorders
- Nausea and sickness

Trusted source study also reports better effects in people that take peppermint oil containing GERD. It's essential, though, that you have never use antacids and peppermint oil concurrently. In reality, it might raise the chance of heartburn.

Ginger Root

For the prevention of nausea, ginger root has traditionally been used. In reality, as short-term steps for pregnancy-linked morning sickness, ginger candy and ginger ale are suggested. Historically, some stomach problems, including heartburn, have been treated with ginger. It is claimed that it produces anti-inflammatory effects. It can decrease the esophagus's swelling and inflammation.

When you consume too high, there are very little ginger root-related side effects. Too much ginger could maybe cause heartburn. Too much ginger could maybe cause heartburn.

Other Herbs

For the care of GERD, a variety of other herbs or botanicals being traditionally used. Even limited scientific data remains to confirm their efficacy. There are among these:

- German Chamomile Flower
- Garden Angelica
- Caraway
- Licorice Root
- Turmeric
- Thistle Milk
- Greater Celandine
- Lemon Balm

Vintage illustration #13_Thristle Milk

17. DYSPEPSIA AND INDIGESTION

Indigestion is also triggered by overeating, eating too much, or having too much greasy or spicy food. Indigestion may also be caused by such mental conditions, including stress or anxiety.

Indigestion in people with the following conditions can be especially common:

- GRED
- Peptic ulcers
- Abnormality of bile ducts or pancreas
- Pancreatitis
- Gastritis
- Stomach cancer
- Gallstones

Although the trademark of indigestion is abdominal discomfort after a meal, other signs can include:

- Mild to unbearable pain or burning in the epigastric, located between the chest bone (lower end) and the navel
- Nausea
- Bloating
- Belching

Since indigestion can, in some cases, signify a more serious condition, it is vital to seek medical assistance if you have symptoms such as:

- Frequent vomiting
- Painful swallowing
- Bloody or black stool
- Weight loss or loss of appetite
- New or worsened heartburn

Indigestion accompanied by sweating, shortness of breath, or pain that radiates to the neck, jaw, or arm.

Demulcents, Bitters, And Carminatives

For indigestion, a stomach disorder, and heartburn, three types of herbs are useful:

- Demulcents, which provide a soothing nature.
- Bitters that induce digestion, and
- Carminatives, which are gas-relieving

Bitter

For indigestion, bitter herbs are useful. The bitter content is considered to improve digestive ability by increasing saliva production while promoting the stomach acid and digestive enzyme. Thus, if stomach acid is poor, bitter herbs become successful. They are not advised if the patient sustains heartburn. The heartburn problem will be intensified in that situation by enhancing already severe stomach acid.

Interestingly, consuming digestive bitters, like an alcoholic beverage just at the end of meals, occurs across South America and Europe. In an ayurvedic medicine system, to boost digestion, a decoction of the bitter herbs can be offered before a meal.

The edible plant Artichoke (Cynara scolymus) has moderate, bitter characteristics. The study has shown that artichoke extracts seem to be beneficial for indigestion. It is particularly useful when bile secretion from the gallbladder isn't adequately induced by inadequate digestion. Medical practitioners normally suggest taking extracts that contain at least 550-1,000 mg/day of cynarin, which is the key active ingredient of Artichoke. As a treatment for indigestion, it is accepted in Europe. Many antioxidants are also found in Artichoke.

Greater celandine named Chelidonium majus study has shown that celandine extract may help alleviate cramping, nausea, and feeling full, more efficiently than a placebo, resulting from indigestion. In the double-blind trial, the dose for six weeks was four mg of chelidonine/capsule with 1or 2 tablets / 3 times a day. Celandine is extremely hazardous for liver disease, and after celandine use, there've been claims of hepatitis-so safety issues are a problem.

For patients that suffer from indigestion, wormwood is often mixed with the carminative herbs. A double-blind clinical trial confirmed that it helped minimize gas and cramping by mixing wormwood with fennel, caraway, and peppermint. While research on natural indigestion remedies is minimal, alternative medicine practitioners may recommend peppermint tea or sipping ginger after a meal to relax the digestive system.

Flavonoids, diterpenes, alkaloids (marrubium), and residues of volatile oils are found in Horehound. Marrubiin, the main active ingredient, and possibly his precursor, premarrubiin, enhance the release of saliva and the release of gastric juices, thereby promoting both the mechanism of appetite and digestion.

Boldo is a historically helpful South American herb for multiple intestinal disorders. This usage may have resulted from its beneficial effect on gastrointestinal infections and the working of the liver. For indigestion and stomach spasms, Germany has permitted its use. One report mixed boldo and other plants and celandine, and Artichoke found that it decreased indigestion severity after two weeks of therapy.

Goldenseal, yarrow, vervain, Yellow dock, and Oregon grape contain bitters used in traditional American medicine. Barberry is a common bitter in Europe that is used for indigestion. Animal testing indicates that these plants promote digestion and alleviate cramps & gas spasms in the intestinal tract.

Picrorhiza, an Indian plant, works like boldo, but human tests have not yet verified its importance.

Blessed thistle, Bitter orange, Centaury, Devil's paw, Dandelion, Elecampane, Bitter melon, Gentian, Juniper, Andrographis, and Prickly ash are among other bitter herbs.

Carminatives (Gas-relieving)

When the indications include belching and gas, carminatives referred to as herbal bitters effectively relieve indigestion because they effectively suppress spasms in the digestive tract. These are possibly very well-studied carminatives and the best recognized and used.

Fennel (Foeniculum vulgare), Caraway (Carum carvi), Peppermint (Mentha piperita), Dbl-blind experiments indicate that mixing peppermint with peppermint, fennel, caraway oil, caraway, and wormwood reduce symptoms of indigestion by minimizing cramping and gas.

Dosage: 3-5 drops of essential oils or 3-5 ml of tincture, taken 2-3 times per day in the water.

And you can crush 2 or 3 teaspoons of seed (caraway, fennel) or peppermint leaves to create tea from herbs, then simmer them in a glass of water for 10 min. An alternate way is to transfer a teaspoon of each to the quart container, let it stay for at least 15 min, low in boiling water, then steadily drink it during the day. Note: if you have heartburn, peppermint will not be beneficial since it relaxes the muscle ring only at the stomach's top.

Ginger

Zingiber officinale has historically been very well regarded as a relief for many gastrointestinal problems, including indigestion, cramping, and gas. It decreases nausea and inflammation and assists with the working of the intestines.

Linden

It has historically been used for indigestion as well. Evidence has indicated the linden flower tea helps those suffering from indigestion, disturbed stomach, or excessive gas. This antispasmodic effect of linden has been validated by research, particularly in the intestines. Linden is not just a carminative but has calming characteristics. By soaking 2-3 teaspoons of the flowers for 15 min, drinking multiple cups every day to alleviate symptoms, you may make Linden tea.

Turmeric

Curcuma longa decreases and relieves inflammation and indigestion. One hundred six patients consuming 500 mg of curcumin four times a day were included in one double-blind study. A placebo and an over the counter anti-indigestion help was given to the control groups. Eighty-seven percent of the participants recorded complete or partial relief of the symptoms after a week (compared with marginally upwards of half of the placebo group). QID was offered to two capsules having 250 mg of turmeric powder in each capsule. Turmeric includes curcumin, which can enhance the work of the gallbladder.

Chamomile

Chamomile decreases inflammation and pain and helps ease the digestive tract (German Chamomile or Matricaria recutita). Chamomile facilitates adequate digestion. The inflammation-and discomfort-reducing characteristics of Chamomile might be beneficial for heartburn-induced discomfort, although there aren't many studies on this. Similarly, Roman Chamomile (Anthemis Nobilis) is being used, but it has not been tested for indigestion.

By applying boiling water to dry chamomile seeds, you may make chamomile tea and soak it for a few minutes. Or, in hot water, you should apply 3-5 ml of chamomile tincture or take 2-3 g 2-4 times per day as tablets.

Lemon balm is also another traditionally utilized carminative herb against indigestion. Lemon balm tea is produced in a sealed container by soaking 2-3 teaspoons leaves around 15 minutes, or you may take 3-5 ml of tincture twice per day.

Artichoke Leaf Extract

Artichoke is rich in antioxidants and antimicrobial properties, which is popular in Mediterranean countries. It has been used to avoid liver damage, lower cholesterol, and relieve dyspepsia.

In a 2015 study, men and women from 17 to 80 years old were monitored who was suffering from stomach pain or uneasiness in the form of nausea or bloating for a period of three months. After taking a supplement blend of artichoke leaf extract and ginger for about two weeks, only the group who consumed the blend felt a reduction in symptoms. Researchers observed at four weeks that in more than 60 percent of cases, the medication decreased indigestion. They theorized that the antispasmodic effects of artichoke leaf extract and its potential to improve bile acid secretion also facilitate gastrointestinal transit, helping relieve bloating and fullness.

Sage

Salvia officinalis is registered for indigestion by Germany but is not indicated for breastfeeding women. The dose is 4-6 g / daily.

Herbs and several popular kitchen spices with which tea may be produced include some carminatives: lavender, coriander, anise, European angelica root, cardamom, rosemary, basil, cinnamon, dill, garlic, oregano, and thyme. Rosemary is also used by European herbal physicians to cure indigestion in the aged.

Due to possible adverse effects, Pennyroyal isn't longer approved for use in patients with indigestion.

Demulcents (Soothing Qualities)

Demulcent herbs minimize inflammation and build a barrier against stomach acid and other irritants in the abdomen.

By containing mucin, a gel-like substance that prevents the symptoms of excessive stomach acid and other adverse irritants, Licorice preserves the digestive tract's lining.26 Deglycyrrhizinated licorice (DGL) is more widely utilized. It is favored since the naturally occurring glycyrrhizin in Licorice has cortisone-like symptoms and can induce water retention, elevated blood pressure, and other issues. However, this portion's absence makes licorice root useful without harming its indigestion helpfulness and dramatically decreases potential side effects. - In general, medical practitioners prescribe 1-2 DGL chewable tabs (250-500 mg), 15 min after foods, and 1-2 hours before bed. DGL is considered to be beneficial against ulcers, although the data is unreliable for indigestion/heartburn.

Slippery Elm has mucilage that may assist heartburn by serving as a shield to acid

Vintage illustration #15_Artichoke

effects on the esophagus. It alleviates swelling, but that is not anti-inflammatory. It's still an antioxidant and helps defend the digestive system against damage caused by free radicals. Generally, medical practitioners prescribe 2-3 capsules containing 400-500 mg, 2-4 times per day. By boiling 1/2-2 g of slippery elm bark in around 3/4 cup of water for 15 min, you can make the tea and cool that for 3-4 cups the day before drinking.

Marshmallow and bladderwrack used as slippery Elm are other demulcents.

Caraway And Peppermint Oil

Research has shown that products consisting of a mixture of enteric-coated peppermint oil and caraway oil can help alleviate indigestion symptoms. This formula is believed to calm the stomach muscles and help food move more easily through the stomach.

18. SINUSITIS AND STUFFY NOSE

Many natural home remedies, steam inhalation, including hydration, and adding a soft, wet towel to the face, will make an individual feel better.

The most frequent source of sinus inflammation is a cold or virus, but a bacterial infection may also source it sometimes.

An individual with sinus congestion can encounter the following, according to the CDC (Centers for Disease Control and Prevention):

- Headaches
- A runny or blocked nose
- Tiredness
- A sore throat
- Coughing

Remedies

There are several home remedies to help alleviate sinus infection that an individual may pursue.

Hydrastis canadensis, widely known as Goldenseal, is often used for sinus infections in the United States since the 18th century. Goldenseal first appeared in 1852 in the U.S Dispensatory and has since held a popular role among the leading herbal medicines.

Thyme

Thymus vulgaris was known primarily as a culinary herb and became popular as an antiseptic in the Middle Ages. Thyme's therapeutic powers derive mainly from its thymol, aromatic oils, and carvacol, producing potent antifungal, antibacterial, expectorant and respiratory relaxant effects. The key therapeutic benefits of volatile oils are directed towards the respiratory system.

Thyme is an outstanding cough remedy that stimulates the immune system as well as simultaneously fights bacteria and viruses. Thyme stimulates phlegm fluidity and facilitates its expulsion.

For curing sinus infection, traditional herbal systems respect diaphoretics. This medicines that facilitate transpiration release waste products and alleviate congestion. A classic example is peppermint. These diaphoretics are better to drink warm. For relieving fever and inflammation, cooling diaphoretics are used. Also, highly antimicrobial are the Chrysanthemum indicum (Chrysanthemum flower) and the Lonicera japonica (Honeysuckle flower). Western diaphoretics include the (Sambucus nigra) Elder flower, (Achillea millefolium) Yarrow flower, and (Eupatorium perfoliatum) boneset leaf.

David Hoffmann, a noted British herbal expert, considers boneset the 'only treatment for relieving the related symptoms.'

Warming the diaphoretics treat these illnesses as well. Using them when chills are the principal symptom. Try the (Ocimum spp.) Basil leaf, which is preferred to suppress mucus within nasal passages in Ayurveda. Bacteria are destroyed by basil, and the immune system is activated. Cinnamon bark (Cinnamomum) is a diaphoretic, very powerful warming, used at a low dose, say 1/2 ounce, or in mixtures of medicinal beverages.

For similar infections, the (Tilia cordata) Linden flower is another diaphoretic utilized extensively in Europe but fairly little in this region. Noted German herbalist Rudolph Weiss states that an outstanding comparative analysis was conducted with (Citrus aurantifolia) Lime blossom against antibiotics in childhood respiratory infections. In reducing the severity and course of the disease, lime blossom tea was much preferable to antibiotics.

Goldenseal

It is the herb's premier anti-infection. Goldenseal's medicinal importance is due to its high Berberine content, which has been proven to have antibacterial and immunostimulatory efficacy. While used for a wide range of ailments, one of garlic's essential activities (Allium sativum) is antimicrobial, owing to the strong sulfur compounds it produces. It has shown that a variety of pathogenic species are greatly inhibited while having no effect on the favorable intestinal flora. Also, garlic has properties that benefit the breathing system.

Sage

Salvia officinalis is a herb rarely used medicinally in the U.S., has an illustrious past among European herbalists. Sage is also used as a herbal gargle for adults, including its strong antimicrobial activity and surprisingly aromatic and slightly pungent flavor.

19. SORE THROAT

Sore throats, particularly in the winter, are one of the most commonly reported illnesses. Usually, these are triggered by infections such as the common cold, flu & strep throat, and although these appear to be very unpleasant, they always go away after a week.

If it is a typical issue in your family, you might like to try building up the body's immune system by using herbal immunostimulants like Echinacea, Siberian Ginseng, and astragalus. Healthy protection against viruses or bacterial infections, which cause sore throats, is a powerful immune system.

Some traditional herbal remedies can give relief. Common ingredients for throat lozenges are menthol, the key fragrance parts of the essential oils of the Japanese mint, peppermint (Mentha ¥piper-ita) and and eucalyptus oil (Eucalyptus spp.) In order to make swallowing less difficult, you may even make your soothing cough drops/teas from licorice root, slippery elm bark, or marshmallow.

Eucalyptus And Menthol

The only U.S FDA approved herbal ingredients to relieve sore throats are eucalyptus oil and menthol, both local anesthetics. Commercial throat lozenges with menthol flavor usually contain menthol around 1 and 10 mg, which might have been obtained from or synthetically produced from mint leaves. Kids below two years should not be given products that contain menthol. In rare circumstances, skin lesions or asthmatic attacks have been caused by items containing menthol added to the skin.

In several cough drops, balms, ointments, nasal inhalers, and mouthwashes, eucalyptus oil is the element. The used amounts in these medications are generally considered secure.

In certain sore-throat lozenges, lemon oil, horehound, hyssop, linden flowers, and different natural ingredients just provide flavoring.

Slippery Elm

Since colonial times, the mucilaginous internal bark of the Ulmus rubra slippery elm has soothed the sore mucous membranes. For more than a century, throat lozenges of Slippery Elm, with their unique sweet scent as well as bland taste, had already stocked United States drugstore shelves.

The bark of this native American tree is collected in early spring. Today, almost entirely in powdered/cut-and-sifted shape, Slippery Elm is available.

In addition to using the bark to cure their sore throats, it was often poulticated on burns, sores, boils, chilblains, and leprosy and syphilis lesions by early immigrants. Bark poultices became the main remedy used during the U.S. Revolution for bullet wounds.

The bark of Slippery Elm has first introduced in the United States in 1820 Pharmacopoeia as an approved medicine for improving mucous membranes. Few pharmacies and health-food stores sell slippery elm lozenges but prefer to create a dense paste of powdered bark of Slippery Elm and honey, shape it into marble-sized balls, then dust every lozenge with dry powder of Slippery Elm. They will be kept in a jar in the freezer forever.

Pour 1 cup of hot water over 1/2 tsp of the fine powder bark to produce a calming drink. Stir till the powder is dissolved and then sip. Drink up to 3 cups a day.

Marshmallow

Althaea officinalis (Marshmallow) roots and leaves, a European native natural-born in North America, often produce mucilage, which can be used to treat sore throats. In situations of a sore throat followed by a dry cough, the German health authorities use leaves and roots preparations to relieve irritated mucous membranes.

The peeled root is known to be of better consistency than the root maintaining its outer bark, and the roots are known to be more effective than the leaves. Marshmallow is provided as teas, tablets, syrups, whole, cut and sifted, and powdered roots.

Pour boiling water (1 cup) over 2 -3 tsp of powdered root/a heaping tbsp of the cut and sifted root, steep about five mins, strain, and taste, to create a good, calming tea. Please take 2 - 3 cups a day.

Marshmallow often activates the immune system slightly. It is usually safe to take both it and Slippery Elm, but its mucilagin content can absorb and therefore decrease the activity of several other drugs taken during that time.

Licorice

The usage of licorice root is decades old for the treatment of sore throats. The root, derived from many members of the pea family of the genus Glycyrrhiza, has an incredibly sweet, musty taste that is due to a compound named glycyrrhizin, a glycoside of triterpene that is 50 times as sweet as sugar.

Licorice is commercially grown in Europe & Asia and is today valued there as a cure for sore throats and also coughs, gastric ulcers, and inflammation.

Put 2 to 3 tbsp of the chopped root in the quart of water to create a decoction and boil till the liquid is decreased to half its original amount. To cure a sore throat, sip around 2 cups each day.

Do not surpass the normal dosage and discontinue usage after four-six weeks. Due to sodium retention and potassium depletion, prolonged use may result in water retention and high blood pressure. Pregnant mothers should not use licorice, persons with cardiac or liver problems, elevated blood pressure, and those using diuretics/digitalis.

20. SPRAINS AND STRAINS

Strains and sprains are different. They have the same signs and effects, but they directly influence various areas of your body.A break or an expansion of the ligament is a sprain. This is the tissue that binds together, which connects bones which cartilage to the joints.A strain is a break in the muscle or tendon or a stretch. One must know what a muscle is, and tendon is a tissue that binds the bone to the muscle. The most frequent sprain occurs in the ankle, while strains in the lower back and hamstring may also occur. They're referring to Grade 1 strain of the muscle when someone says, "I strained my muscle," It takes days or weeks for them to recover. A Grade 2 strain is caused by additional muscle fibers tearing, creating additional pain and discomfort. Such strains need medical attention and can take a few months to be 100 percent cured. A Grade 3 strain is extreme because there is a rupture of the muscle or tendon. Often, to reconnect the muscle or tendon, you can require surgery and the healing period is many months.

Rosmarinus Officinalis (Rosemary)

This is a warm herb that helps with healing, pain, and inflammation by bringing blood flow to the region. Inflammation is not a derogatory term. It's a soothing mechanism that our body has naturally. Instead of just getting rid of it, use herbs that aid recovery so that it eventually goes out. Use in a soak or compress.

Arnica Homoeopathic

It's the first thing you can aim for, as this is a homeopathic cure. Inflammation, bruising, and pains are aided. This is the Arnica type only that is perfect for internal use.

Cream / Oil Arnica (Arnica Montana)

Typically, this one is produced with the Arnica herb and is really very quick to produce. You're not supposed to apply it on the skin that is broken. Use it when needed.

Symphytum Officinale (Comfrey)

This strong herb is perfect for tissue (as well as bone) healing. Using it in a soak or a compress.

Officinalis Calendula (Calendula)

This vivid, warm herb helps inflammation and discomfort. For broken skin, it is safe. Use it in herbal infused oil, compress, or soak.

Lavandula Officinalis (Lavender)

An essential oil and herb for inflammation and pain. Usage of soaked, compressed, herbal infused, or essential oils. A 25 percent dilution rate with Lavender EO, 25 drops/one teaspoon, is safe for acute use. It's for adults.

For children below 12, 2 drops/tsp (2%) for acute use is fine.

Although Lavender essential oil is considered safe for "neat" application, there is still a threat over time of sensitization. That implies for the 1st, 2nd, or 3rd time you might not react, but if you choose to use it neatly ... you might notice for you break out in hives or even have a significant reaction. Just be safe.

Aches And Pain Blend:

- 1/4 cup of Comfrey Dry Leaves
- 1/4 cup of Calendula Flowers Dried
- 1/4 Cup of Rosemary Leaves Dried
- 1/4 cup of dry buds of Lavender
- 1/2-1 cup of Magnesium or Himalayan pink salt

Instructions and usage:

- Add all the ingredients to a big canning jar, then hand mix thoroughly.
- In 1 quart of boiling water, utilizing a 1/4 to 1/2 cup herb mix.
- Steep for 15 mins.
- Soak the kitchen towel in infusion as a compress and put over the sprain/strain. Twenty minutes to rest and swap out and keep things warm.
- When soaked-add infusion either to a foot bath or, if necessary, full.
- Repeat throughout the day several times.

21. SKIN

For centuries, herbal remedies have persisted and been used to cure several conditions varying from slight stomach discomfort to cancer. Recent studies confirm the usage of herbs in the cure of multiple medical conditions.

Dr. Doris Day, a dermatologist at the N.Y. U. Medical Center in Manhattan, advises that "If I were to select just one natural cure for the treatment of skin disorders, aloe vera would be my number one preference. It has been commonly accepted as a special curing plant." Aloe Vera is used as a skin softener & moisturizer in its pure form.

The gel has been used for decades to speed up wound recovery and fluid inside the plants. Not only does it enhance regeneration, but it also acts as topical pain relief. "Unfortunately, several of the items in the markets containing aloe vera may not have ample concentration of the substance in them to render them safe," Dr. Day says. Some reputable tests have shown that aloe vera is very effective in curing psoriasis, a relatively common disease that contributes to itchy skin and scalp red scaly patches.

Arnica

Arnica flower by tropical preparations is extremely useful for wound curing. As an analgesic (pain reliever), anti-inflammatory, and antiseptic cream, it is successful. Dr. Day also states that "this procedure is prescribed regardless of trauma or surgeries for bruising and swelling." It is also effective in speeding up the recovery of simple skin abrasions, bug bites, and soothing joint discomfort. The German government has licensed the usage of arnica for the healing of wounds.

Calendula

This flower is often referred to as the common marigold and has a strong history of success in treating bruises, burns, skin disorders, cuts and rashes. The German health authorities also approved its usage for topical treatment of badly healing wounds and some forms of skin ulcers. There are also compresses produced of helpful calendula tea. In order to relieve sore lesions in the mouth, tea is sometimes used as a mouthwash.

For decades, both the leaves and roots of Comfrey were used to enhance the treatment of cuts and bruises. It has also proven effective for the prevention of rashes as an anti-inflammatory. When added to the skin over the accident site, it is believed to facilitate closed fractures recovery. While topical usage of the roots or leaves is healthy, application over damaged skin may contribute to toxicity. Therefore, it should not be applied for more than three days in a row. Tea made from comfrey leaves is also helpful, but it should not be exceeding three cups a day.

Tea Tree
A tall evergreen growing in Asia and Australia is the tea tree. The leaves were used as an antiseptic for decades and were used as a disinfectant during World War I. More recently, oil has been extracted from the leaves to treat wounds, bug bites and other common skin issues. Both fungus and bacteria were shown to kill the oil. The oil is sold in supermarkets without a prescription and may be refined under different circumstances, if appropriate. Tea tree oil can be poisonous and can never be given orally.

Chamomile
It was used for the management of numerous medical conditions for centuries. For slight stomach, upset, dried and fresh flowers rendered into a tea is used as an oral scrub to treat gingivitis and sore mouth lesions, and topically to promote wound healing and treat moderate skin conditions, such as hives, itchy lesions, and sunburn.

Cayenne
This spicy red pepper has been used for a number of medical conditions, such as stomach ulcers, high blood pressure, poor circulation, skin and lungs infections. In order to optimize anti-inflammatory and antibacterial effects, there are several formulations that blend capsaicin with other herbal ingredients.
Capsaicin has been found to deplete the substance-P from nerve ends, which, according to Dr. Day, allows it an appropriate pain reliever. The discomfort can initially escalate, or there could be a burning feeling due to substance-P release, which is normally temporary.
Ineffectively treating skin disorders, several natural medicines are useful. Dr. Day

Vintage illustration #16_Chamomile

insists that if the individual using them is allergic to any of the active compounds, such herbal remedies can cause adverse reactions. When a skin disorder continues or signs become worse, it is advised to see a doctor.

22. WOUNDS

Open wounds are indeed a nightmare; they are not only painful and messy, but they still require months to fully recover. They leave, not to overlook, a lasting stain on your skin. As if this is not enough, one has to make sure that perhaps the wound is protected from being poisoned, which speeds down the process of healing. It may or may not encourage the wound to heal by adding various commercial ointments to the wound, but some kitchen items may work wonders. Due to their medicinal powers, some of the ingredients widely used in edible delicacies serve as healers or ideal cure. Are. These natural remedies will help you to disinfect your wound to make sure it's dis-infected. To get the greatest performance, make sure to use them daily. Please notice that these ingredients function well for mild wound therapies. Please resort to treatment under observation in the event of serious injuries.

To ensure fast recovery and avoid infection, here are a few home remedies.

Garlic
Garlic has been noted for its antimicrobial and antibiotic abilities, which can help stop bleeding quickly, minimize pain, and encourage healing. Currently, garlic often strengthens the normal protection of the body against infection. Just add some crushed garlic cloves to it if the wound is bleeding.

Turmeric
A natural antiseptic and antibiotic product that has been used for its therapeutic purposes for years is the humble kitchen spice. According to research reported in the journal Molecular And Cellular Biochemistry, curcumin in Turmeric helps improve wound healing by modulating collagen. Add Turmeric to the wound if the wound bleed and the bleeding will cease instantly. Drink a glass of milk with Turmeric every night to recover fully before going to bed.

Aloe Vera
The analgesic, anti-inflammatory, and relaxing effects of Aloe Vera promote the phase of recovery. In reality, there are phytochemicals in the gel that help alleviate pain and decrease inflammation. Break open the leaves of the aloe vera and

Vintage illustration #17_Onion

remove the gel. Place the gel on the wound & allow it to dry. With warm water, rinse the region and pat dry with a towel.

Coconut Oil

Owing to its moisturizing, antibacterial, and anti-inflammatory effects, coconut oil helps relieve pain and keeps illnesses at bay. Actually, coconut oil also helps prevent scarring. One needs to add this oil with a clean cloth to the infected region and cover it. At least 2 to 3 times a day, re-apply the coconut oil.

Coconut oil tends to alleviate pain and keep infections at bay.

Onion

Onion does have an antimicrobial component called allicin, which prevents the wound of infection. In a mixer, mix the onion and honey and create a paste. Directly apply to the wound to speed up the process of healing.

CONCLUSION

Throughout history, natural resources have become a significant source of medicinal agents, and modern medicine tends to focus on traditional knowledge for human disease care. Numerous indigenous medicine systems have well-accepted the therapeutic power of herbs. In addition to their medicinal application, plants are preventers of infections and are often used as nutritional, cosmetics, supplements, and combat obesity. In contrast to medicinal plants, the interest of developed countries is distinct from that of developing countries. Developed countries are hunting for leads to therapeutic plant medicines. In contrast, emerging countries will prefer to provide cheaper herbal formulations because they cannot afford the long road of pure compound drug exploration.

Herbal medicine is the central focus of complementary and holistic medicine, which has acquired growing popularity across the globe in recent years and is steadily streaming towards integration into the established healthcare systems. Herbalists prefer to use extracts from sections of plants, such as the leaves or roots, assuming that plants are sensitive to natural stresses and therefore establish tolerance to hazards such as reactive oxygen species, microbial attack, and radiations, offering protective phytochemicals for use in herbalism.

ABOUT THE AUTHOR

Tamaya Kawisenhawe was born in Santa Barbara and earned her master's degree in botany at Claremont Graduate University (California).

After becoming a naturopathic and acupuncturist, she moved to Portland where she lives with her husband and two daughters. She has worked with medicinal herbs for more than 15 years.

Now, she decides to share and spread her passion and knowledge with others, running seminars all around the country.

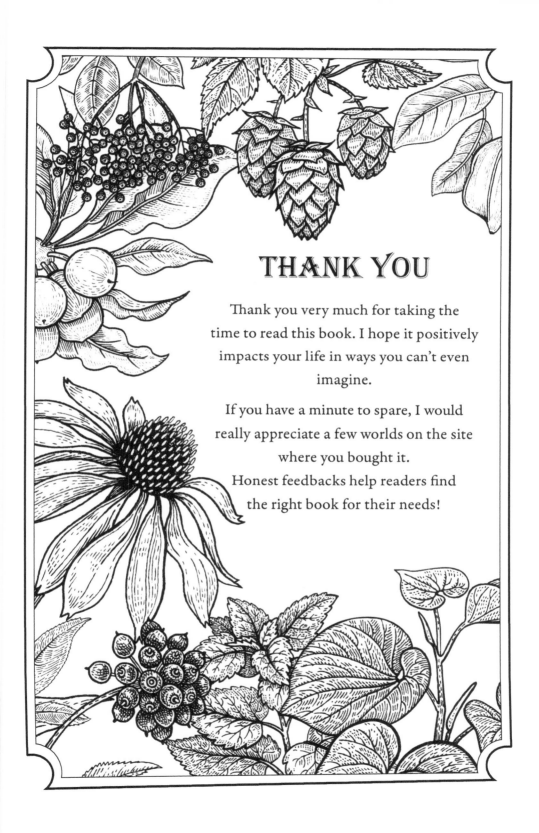

THANK YOU

Thank you very much for taking the time to read this book. I hope it positively impacts your life in ways you can't even imagine.

If you have a minute to spare, I would really appreciate a few worlds on the site where you bought it.
Honest feedbacks help readers find the right book for their needs!